Fr. Ron,

I hope you enjoy

this as much as I did.

Paul Sullivan

FACING PAIN, FINDING HOPE

FACING PAIN, FINDING HOPE

A PHYSICIAN EXAMINES
PAIN, FAITH, AND
THE HEALING
STORIES OF JESUS

DANIEL HURLEY, MD

LOYOLAPRESS.

CHICAGO

LOYOLAPRESS.

3441 N. ASHLAND AVENUE
CHICAGO, ILLINOIS 60657
WWW.LOYOLABOOKS.ORG

Cover and interior design by Gloria Chantell

Library of Congress Cataloging-in-Publication Data
Hurley, Daniel (Daniel John), 1957-
  Facing pain, finding hope : a physician examines pain, faith, and the healing stories of Jesus / Daniel Hurley.
     p. cm.
  Includes bibliographical references and index.
  ISBN 0-8294-1780-X (alk. paper)
  1. Pain—Religious aspects—Christianity. 2. Consolation—Biblical teaching. 3. Bible. N.T. Gospels—Criticism, interpretation, etc. I. Title.
BT732.7.H87 2005
248.8'6—dc22

2005010669

Printed in the United States of America
05 06 07 08 09 10 M-V 10 9 8 7 6 5 4 3 2 1

To Mom, Dad, Mike, and Mary

CONTENTS

Fear crackles like fire in every life, fed by the uncertainties that are a constant part of people and events. Small wonder that we dream universally of desert islands, of quiet safe places where we might catch our breath for a moment. But there are no such islands, not for any of us. There is only life, unfolding quite mysteriously and with ever-present challenge even in the most commonplace existences.
Eugene C. Kennedy, *The Pain of Being Human*

ACKNOWLEDGMENTS

First, I would like to thank my dear longtime friend Patrice Tuohy, a professional writer and editor, for putting her faith in me from the very beginning and giving me the chance to bring this book into existence. I want to thank my editor Vinita Wright for her kind, gentle guidance through this first effort of mine to hone a manuscript into a book. She made it very easy for me, and I am truly grateful. I would like to thank all those at Loyola Press who have given me the opportunity and freedom to speak from my spiritual heart and my medical head. I especially want to thank Jim Manney and Matthew Diener for their words of encouragement and guidance, along with Michelle Halm and Mary Edsey for their enthusiasm.

Going back a ways, I have to thank my four high school English teachers, who truly set me on the path of loving literature and writing. Paul Zook, Tom Meyer (deceased), John Hussong, and Jim Cahill all taught me at St. Xavier High School in Cincinnati, Ohio. I am indebted to their dedication and great skills as teachers in both challenging and inspiring me long beyond my days in their classes so many years ago.

I must thank all those priests and nuns who taught me and ministered to me throughout my life in Catholic schools and attending Catholic services. In many ways, their faith and words were God's own as I grew in faith. Most important, I must thank my two college chaplains at the Harvard Catholic Student Center, Father Tom Powers and Sister Evelyn Ronan. They are two of the most wonderful people I have ever known, and I thank God for sending them into my life at such an important time. They became my spiritual parents when I left home and showed up in Cambridge, Massachusetts, at that first Mass of freshman year at Harvard. They have since remained treasured friends and guides, blessings to me beyond words.

I want to thank all my friends and teachers from across the years. They have each been God's unique presence in my life. I thank all the doctors, nurses, and therapists who have contributed to my medical training each step of the way, even to this very day. And I thank all the patients who have entrusted their lives for a time to my care.

I specifically thank my partners, staff, and patients at the Chicago Institute of Neurosurgery and Neuroresearch where I have been practicing since 1995 for allowing me a mini-sabatical to put the finishing edits on the book. Thanks also to Eastern Point Retreat House, a special place on the New England coast, for providing me quiet and inspiration over the years on this journey.

Finally, I thank my parents and my brother and sister. My family has loved me beyond measure in all aspects of my life. They have gifted me with their faith; have lavished on me devotion, tolerance, and support; and have given me so much more of themselves than I have ever been able to return. I thank you, Mom, Dad, Mary, and Michael.

Of course, I thank You, God, for the gift of this life, the gifts of these people, and the gift of this chance to write about You.

1

"TELL ME YOUR STORY."

A Pain Specialist Searches
for the Sacred

The waiting room was so full of patients, it looked like an airport on a snowy day. I walked through to the back of the clinic to begin my morning schedule. It was a multiphysician office, so I didn't know which of those people were waiting to see me. I did know that each had a story of pain to tell, a history of suffering.

I had just come from the hospital chapel, where I had gone after making rounds through the wards. Kneeling there, knowing I had a heavy workload with two meetings in the afternoon, I wondered how others were facing their day. Some were waking up to another day of tormenting pain. Some had risen at 4:00 a.m. to get to the hospital for a surgery they very much feared but needed. Others had to muster the energy to go to dialysis or chemotherapy. In some households, spouses were facing the likelihood that this would be the last day they saw their husbands or wives, or if they saw them again it would be in intensive care fighting for their lives.

> *They brought to him all who were sick with various diseases and racked with pain, those who were possessed, lunatics, and paralytics, and he cured them. . . . At the sight of the crowds, his heart was moved with pity for them because they were troubled and abandoned, like sheep without a shepherd. (Matthew 4:24; 9:36)*

I had earlier walked slowly around the chapel, past the stations of the cross. I looked at the crucifix and saw the suffering God. *What do I learn from you, Lord? What do I bring from here over to my office where your suffering people wait? The "good news" that we must die first as a grain of wheat planted in the ground, or that we must pick up our crosses and walk with you? Or the "good news" that your yoke is easy and your burden is light?*

I rode the elevator down to the clinic, praying that I could somehow bridge the gap between Jesus' life and ours, between the miracles we read about in the Bible and the miracles we pray for every day. When I reached the exam rooms, my medical assistant told me the first patient was ready in room one and that it seemed like a tough case. "And she talks a lot, Doctor, so don't get us all behind now with the very first one." I don't think Jesus had appointment times, do you?

One Story of Many

Joan was an attractive thirty-six-year-old woman, with an athletic form and a slightly anxious, though pleasant, demeanor. "Doctor, I don't know if you can help me. I've been so many places already. I didn't want to come today, but a friend of mine had been here and had done well. She suggested I come in, too. I checked out your Web site, and I figured maybe you'd be a good person to try, though I'm really not sure."

"Why don't you explain your situation, and I'll let you know whether there is anything I can suggest. If I can't, maybe I'll know someone who can, okay?"

So she proceeded to tell me her story: three and a half years of mysterious, persistent abdominal and pelvic pain. It had started innocently enough with left thigh pain, which she thought was just a muscle strain, having just returned to running after delivering her second child.

She tried stretching, massage, and even acupuncture with someone a friend had recommended. The pain didn't really go away but shifted from her thigh into a deep area in her pelvis and lower abdomen. She went to her gynecologist, who couldn't find any problems that might have resulted from her pregnancy or delivery. She was sent to a gastrointestinal specialist who diagnosed her with irritable bowel syndrome and started her on some medicine and an altered diet. Neither worked, and her pain was, instead, getting worse and becoming much more crampy and debilitating.

After a year, she went back to her gynecologist, who took some more tests and felt that perhaps there were some signs of uterine dysplasia (abnormal appearance of the growth pattern of the cells). In addition, there now seemed to be signs of dysfunctional uterine bleeding. Given the length of time the pain had persisted, the lack of response to treatment, and concerns over the abnormal bleeding and biopsy results, the doctor suggested a hysterectomy.

That was a bit stunning to both Joan and her husband. They had never planned a big family but were hoping for perhaps a third child in a couple of years. Nevertheless, with the pain so intense and persistent, and the fear of something more serious being the cause, the couple agreed to the surgery. Two years later she came to see me.

Even after the acute recovery from the surgery itself, she was surprised to find how fatigued and weak she remained for several months afterward. But more frightening to her was that her pain wasn't dramatically decreased. After eight months had gone by and she was still in pain, she became depressed. She agreed to take antidepressants, but combining those with the pain pills she was on already made her feel mentally dulled. The narcotic side effect of constipation caused additional abdominal and pelvic pain, only confusing the picture as to whether she should take more or less of the medicine.

Searching the Internet, she'd read that back problems could manifest in unusual locations, such as wrapping around the abdomen or with deep aching in the pelvis. She went to a specialist at the university hospital. The MRI of her spine did in fact reveal a small disc abnormality at the level in her vertebrae that might possibly correlate with the location of her pain, so physical therapy and a cortisone injection were ordered. Initially, she did perceive some relief with this approach, but it was short-lived.

Further tests on her spine were ordered, and further injections were given, which again led to a transient abatement of her symptoms. It was at least more of a response than she had experienced with anything else. Unfortunately, the relief could not be sustained, and in the end she was left with her pain and a tough decision. The spine doctors were suggesting back surgery to remove the suspected offending disc and replace it with a fusion. It was that, or live with it. That is when she made the appointment to see me, and it had taken her about five weeks to get in.

"That's basically how I got here. Can you make me well again? I really don't want to have to go through another surgery. They can't tell me it will get rid of my pain for certain. I was desperate the first time, and afraid I might have cancer. But, now . . . I mean, I can't stand this pain—it's totally changed my life—but a surgery on the spine, the risks of paralysis or my bladder not working right afterward. I can't face that. Do you possibly have any other ideas on how I can get well?"

What could I possibly say or do to give her a sense of hope and of options? *Lord, it seemed your miracles were so quick: a touch of your hands, a blessing and a command, a brush against a tassel. And the illnesses were gone. I don't have that miracle wand.*

Where to Begin

I write from the perspective of a physician dealing with people who suffer pain and disabilities. My specialty is called Physical Medicine and Rehabilitation—Physiatry, or PM&R for short. I have been the caregiver to those who often felt no hope of recovery: the permanently paralyzed or brain injured, the amputees, those born with cerebral palsy or deformities, those suffering from degenerative muscle and nerve diseases, and those suffering the disease of pain—pain from an endless list of causes. After an emotional struggle during medical school, I gave up the image of being a towering neurosurgeon to enter instead my relatively obscure specialty. I chose, without quite knowing it, the world of suffering.

I happen to be Catholic. I was born to devoutly Catholic parents. Their love, self-sacrifice, generosity, faith, and commitment led me to trust the religion into which I was born. I was blessed with guides and mentors all along the way, and I grew up with a desire to search out lessons given to us as gifts in the Bible, and most specifically through the words of Jesus in the Gospels. Though I am not one to memorize and formally quote Scripture, I do seek wisdom and guidance from those ancient writings and am amazed, albeit sometimes confused, by God's communications to us through Bible stories.

I recognize that all the Scripture writings were written by real human beings, at specific moments in history. Christians believe these words to be inspired, but we accept that, for instance, not every single word or lesson Christ spoke during his time on earth was recorded. Thus, by definition, we read in the Bible only part of the story of God's loving relationship with God's creation. The rest we must gain through genuine and truthful searching, prayer, and learning from the continued workings of the Holy Spirit through history. If nothing else, Christians struggle each day to discern how we are to apply God's words to the limitless variety of events and challenges that we encounter.

In the past seventeen years of seeing patients in practice, and the eight years of medical training prior to that, I have come to recognize in my patients and their plights some of the familiar individuals in the Gospel stories. I have tried to understand the ways Jesus cared for his own patients and, thus, the instruction he offers each of us in how to handle illness, pain, suffering, and challenge. These healing stories in the Gospels have come to take on a kind of archetypal quality. I return to them again and again as I try to unravel the mysteries of faith and suffering that show up in the people who ask for my help.

When someone like Joan walks into my office, I try first of all to broaden her understanding of pain: its definition, its mechanisms, and its impact on her life. This opens up more possibilities for treatment and for coping with a problem that, often, we cannot simply make go away. It also allows me to get to know the patient, and the patient to gain some trust in me.

I want my patients to be aware of how their mental states affect their tolerance of pain, and how what goes on in their lives and environments influences how they see their conditions and their options for healing. Do they dare step outside the box that has defined them thus far? Do they see where anger plays a role? Are there hidden factors that somehow lead them to hold onto their sick roles, or do others suspect that they are possibly even faking their symptoms? Do they dare ask for help when they are beaten? And can they really see who they are as persons anymore when they have been defined by illness for so long?

My hope is that, through my various encounters with the patient, an educational process takes place, allowing knowledge and understanding to grow. I also hope to strengthen the connections among everyone involved in the healing process.

There is rarely enough time for the doctor or patient to share their thoughts freely, nor is it always appropriate to do so in a hospital or medical office setting. This is especially true in regard to the special and intimate subject of spirituality. Spirituality is one facet of care that doesn't get much attention in the average medical interaction, even though studies have shown that the vast majority of patients and doctors believe spirituality to be an important aspect of healing and coping.

This book is the result of my own struggle to connect my work as a physician with the ultimate healing work of Jesus in the Gospels. I present those rich, ageless stories along with composites of patients whom I have encountered over the years. None of the patients in this book is an actual identifiable person, so if you happen to have been a patient of mine and think you recognize yourself, rest assured that it is only because so many others have similar stories. No individual patient is presented as him- or herself. The only factual contemporary characters are my brother Michael and my two friends Julie and Patrick.

As for Joan back in my clinic office, her problem was not going to be easy to solve. I agreed with her that the decision to go ahead with surgery was a difficult one. As I tell almost all my patients, it is hard to "try" surgeries. You try medicines and therapies. You *get* surgeries. The more aggressive the treatment, the more cautious you need to be in order to weigh the costs. Doctors know that their best efforts have been blunted before. Patients have tried so many things already. Joan had been to many doctors and tried many therapies and solutions. We had to decide with care what the next step should be.

In the chapters to come, we will begin where Joan was left: at the point of facing the reality of her pain, even as she sought to eradicate it. We will then explore the healing stories of the Gospels, in which people live in pain and fight to hope for something better. We will watch their encounters with Jesus and see what choices they make concerning not only their medical problems but their whole lives.

I explore only a handful of Jesus' miracles. But the goal is to stretch those stories a bit and, in so doing, to stretch ourselves, so that we can discover possibilities and graces that we may not have been aware of before. God is eternal and not limited by time and circumstance. Likewise, Jesus is a doctor with no rushed appointment schedule and no need of malpractice insurance. We can talk to him freely and ask him any questions. The real issue, however, is how we will answer the questions he poses to us.

Before getting directly into the Gospel healing stories and evaluating the actions of our Lord and his "patients," let us touch first on some of the issues and questions I hear from patients every day in my office. There is the issue of "just living with" pain; there is also the presence of anger, the question of the legitimacy of complaints, and the desperation that looks further and further for relief.

2

"YOU MEAN I HAVE TO LIVE WITH THIS?"

The First Reality in the Journey Forward

Like shadowy Homeric spirits of the dead, chronic pain patients tend to move in an in-between realm: they clearly are not well, but their malady will not let us see them as absolutely sick. . . . It is easy to entertain this thought until one day chronic pain hits you with its invisible fist, like a knife in the back that the doctors cannot find. Suddenly nothing looks the same. It is as if the world has abruptly and completely changed, turned sinister, even evil, but no one knows except you.

David B. Morris, *The Culture of Pain*

As in the story of Joan shared earlier, patients in pain have a tremendously difficult time when trying to convey to physicians, and sometimes to their families, the extent and nature of their pain. They can become terribly frustrated when trying to convince me of just exactly how bad their pain really is. Listen to a few examples of what five different patients have said to me. Believe me, they speak for the rest.

"So, you're telling me I just have to live with this. You're telling me this is all in my head. I just have to take pain medicines for the rest of my life. You're saying there's no surgery for this, that there's nothing wrong. How can the MRI not show something? I don't believe that this is just some 'degenerative condition that everyone has,' that 'it's just part of getting older,' that I should have to be in so much pain. I don't think you understand, Doctor, what I mean by pain. This is not just some soreness or some muscle problem. I know what that feels like. And I can tolerate pain. I had a gunshot wound once, and I could handle that. I had a piece of glass stuck in my arm, and I handled that better than the doctor did."

"I have given birth to three children without an epidural. That hurt, but not like this. I can't sit; I can't walk; I can't stand; I can't even stay lying down for very long. I never sleep for more than two hours at a time. Don't even ask when the last time I had sex was. I don't pick up the baby because I'm afraid I'll drop her from the pain. I haven't woken up a day in my life for the past three and a half years when I didn't feel the pounding, tightening pain. And it only gets worse through the day, with shooting and burning."

"I'm horrible to live with, my wife and kids will tell you that. We have no money because the insurance company cut me off, and I don't get disability because their doctor said I could work. How the heck am I supposed to work like this! I can't even drive to get to a job. What are they going to have me do? I can't do anything all day, even at home. Nobody can find out why I'm in so much pain. All these doctors and specialists and insurance people—I'd like to see them go through what I go through for just one day. Hell, now they act like it's all in my head. It's not in my head, it's in my back! So I'm supposed to just live with this? Bullshit!"

"I am so tired of this pain. I just want my life back. I feel like I'm not even me anymore. I can't believe that God wants me to live my life like this. I feel so badly that I can't do anything for anyone anymore. I used to cook and clean all the time, help my kids with their homework, be on their school committees, and go to every one of their games. We would have the neighbors and friends over all the time; I loved to entertain. Now it is impossible to even think of such things. I am exhausted and miserable all the time. This is not living."

"I sometimes wonder whether God is testing me, or punishing me, by letting me go through this. I haven't asked for much, but it seems like if anything can go wrong with my health, it does. Other people go through their surgeries and they're up and around so fast and back into their normal routines. They told me, 'Oh it's nothing, you'll feel great. It will be like you never had a problem in the first place.' I don't know. Something either went wrong with my treatment or they haven't found what's really wrong. I don't think I'm that much of a wimp or crybaby, but I just can't take this much longer."

Sound familiar? As a doctor specializing in back and neck problems, spinal disorders, headaches, and other orthopedic and neurologic conditions such as carpal tunnel syndrome, shoulder and knee injuries, hip arthritis, strokes, head injuries, spinal cord injuries, amputations, burns—to name just the familiar ones—I can assure you that I have been on the receiving end of countless verbal complaints like the ones above. Sometimes the anger and frustration are aimed at me. Other times they are aimed at the list of prior doctors or at the insurance company or an employer. Occasionally a family member gets to bear the brunt of the lashing. Sometimes it's the system, the world, the general way things are. Secretly, for many of us, our ultimate and true target is God.

How Do We Bear an Inescapable Burden?

There is no end to the varieties of pain each of us must endure and thus no end to the moments during which we are forced to respond to its presence. We all dread the thought of a painful trauma such as a car accident, plane crash, or fire. We fear being attacked and assaulted by some robber or intruder; being stabbed, shot, or beaten. Even less catastrophic injuries such as broken legs, torn ligaments, cuts, or dental work intimidate us to some extent.

There are some, however, who must deal with what is simply termed chronic pain, though it is anything but simple in its nature and impact. Sometimes surgeries do not work their miracles but instead leave disappointment and torment. Tragic misfortunes, one after another, befall some unlucky souls. Others are burdened with bodies and genetics that seem to make them prone to, and plagued by, an unbelievable number of diseases and organ malfunctions. Meanwhile, these same people have friends or relatives who live anything but healthy lifestyles—smoking, drinking, and eating all the "wrong," "bad" things—and yet they carry on merrily into their nineties.

Some people will be forced to go through their lives with long-term scars, permanent disabling conditions, or congenital deformities. Others will languish in the long-drawn sadnesses of life, the losses that cannot be replaced, the dreams forever abandoned, the chances missed, the disappointments and disillusionments, and the realizations that come too late to right a wrong. This wondrous gift of life, from a merciful, loving God can then seem so dry and meaningless. Are we unappreciative creatures when we sink to such dullness? Even as we acknowledge the power of positive thinking and presence of true grace, our human spirit can endure only so much before it is beaten down from its long-suffering.

Then comes the broken spirit and the further laments, such as these:

- "I am too young for this pain, Doctor. I shouldn't have to live like this. There has got to be something you can do. I want to get back to what I used to do, how I used to be. I just want to be able to hang out with my kids. I just want to play golf."

- "I would be happy to be able to walk to the store, to cook dinner, to go to church. I just wish I could walk again."

- "I am so alone. I feel so guilty. I cannot live without my husband."

- "How could God have taken my son?"

- "I am so tired all the time. I cannot even see the future. This is not living."

Life for couples can change quite drastically when one of them is afflicted with pain. For the husband or wife suffering in illness, direct, blinding pain may fill every day. For the spouse, the intimate experience of living with someone made different by his or her pain affects a marriage now also made different—for better or for worse, and seemingly only worsening.

Does our God just allow us to drift through life as it has been dealt us? Are we then to feel guilty for being like the Israelites who wandered out into the desert with Moses, complaining bitterly when they were lost, hungry, and tired? Are we like those skeptics in the crowd who demanded a sign of Jesus? Are we not also like Thomas, who kept in check any personal celebration of Jesus' rising from the dead, questioning the promises and testimonials of his fellow disciples? "Show me the money first" is perhaps the modern vernacular for his response.

Pain is so common and mundane that we tend to consider it part of normal life. It is often not tied to an ultimate, gallant struggle to die a dignified death in the face of a terminal cancer, a major heart attack, or a rare incurable disease. We cannot gauge pain by numbers, as with glucose levels in diabetes or blood counts in anemia or leukemia. It slowly and stealthily eats away at the vibrancy of life, dulling it into inactivity and drugged oblivion. But even in diseases such as diabetes, anemia, leukemia, congestive heart failure, and a plethora of others, the invisible aspects of pain and exhaustion are much of the true burden.

In the collective mind-set of the medical profession, and even in society at large, there has been a fairly blatant distinction made between the pain and suffering associated with malignancy or terminal illnesses and that which accompanies "benign," "non-life-threatening" disorders such as arthritis, headache, back problems, or mental illness. The widespread stigma of, and resistance to, prescribing high-dose narcotic pain medicine, even in situations of death and dying, has only recently been overcome. Pain specialists are now finally being more aggressive in the treatment of pain for those with so-called benign chronic disorders. I contend that some of these so-called benign chronic disorders are so deeply debilitating that they are life-threatening in their own right—they are the cause of slow deaths that drag on over years and years, affecting families as much as patients. In poorly managed situations, addiction to the very drugs and medications used in treatment is itself a form of death that is just as slow.

Headache and back pain rank first and second, respectively, as the primary reasons people see their doctors for pain. I see thousands of patients a year with such problems. In my consultations, many times late in the evenings, in darkened hospital rooms, I hear story after story of patients with years, almost lifetimes, of disabling spinal disorders or constant headaches—such a monstrosity this thing we call pain, which surrounds the very space in which we live, think, concentrate, plan, and remember. The desperation I hear from so many people is overwhelming. "Doctor, if you don't do something about this pain soon, I'm about ready to put a bullet through my head. I just don't care anymore. I can't take this."

This is a delicate moment, and sometimes doctors don't have the curative, relieving answers. We cannot lie in order to protect ourselves, to save our own images as great, knowledgeable healers. We cannot succumb to the temptation of rescuing patients from their misery by making false, grandiose claims. Yet we must always provide some aspect of hope. What happens when there is no easy answer?

One Image to Describe Pain

There are some situations in which people don't "feel" pain from an obviously painful trauma, such as a broken bone or an amputation. We hear heroic stories of mothers or fathers, soldiers or accident victims performing amazing acts after having sustained major injuries themselves. We hear of athletes who play full games after incurring broken ankles, ribs, or jaws in the opening minutes of the contest. Do these people "feel" their pain, or are the signals somehow delayed? The body does have biologic mechanisms to enhance survival in hostile environments, and one of the most well-known is its ability to instantly produce morphinelike substances of enkephalins and endorphins. In acute-pain situations, these internal chemicals block the full brunt of pain in order for the individual to focus on actions for survival or for the survival of others. In chronic pain, however, this system loses its power, and other processes act almost in reverse, causing phenomena such as "windup," wherein early limited pain becomes compounded as it becomes more chronic. This makes the battle to handle pain during the suffering phase that much more challenging.

The tough thing about pain is that it's multilayered. It is tied to personality, psychology, and social context as much as, or more than, it is tied to biology. There is a very helpful simple image in medicine describing this layered nature of pain. It is that of a set of four concentric circles. The smallest, most inner circle is the actual tissue-damaging event, or in psychological situations, the emotional or stressful traumatic event. Physically, this could be something as simple as stubbing a toe or burning a finger, to breaking a leg or getting a cut, to much more severe major trauma. It could be a tumor pressing on a nerve. It could be the news visually or audibly that someone has just died.

The second, slightly larger circle is that of neural sensation of pain, or what in medical terms is called "nociception." Specialized nerve endings register painful stimuli and send them up the nerves into the spinal cord via electrically propagated impulses. In a very simple description of what occurs, most of these signals travel up the spine in a specific bundle of wires within the larger cable that is the spinal cord itself. Many reflexes and modulations can occur even at this level, but for our purposes, this connection from site of injury to the top of the spinal column is the second circle of pain.

Once the signals reach the deep inner core of the brain stem and proceed to the part of the brain called the thalamus, we are in the third circle of pain in this model. It is at this point that the brain first becomes aware that a painful event has occurred. The thalamus is the clearinghouse for all these signals, and it is from here that word is sent to all parts of the nervous system that something painful has happened. A general alarm has been sounded. The exact location of the pain is identified if that is possible (as opposed to vague pain, which is hard to pinpoint, as we all know). Protective reflexes are set in motion, such as withdrawal of a hand from a hot stove, the instant closing of the eyelids to brightness, the hunching of the neck and shoulders to a blow on the head or a sudden loud noise. Meanwhile, signals are also sent out to judgment centers.

This brings us to the fourth and largest circle of pain, that which we call suffering. It dwarfs the three inner circles. This fourth circle encompasses the experience of pain within the context of all events, memories, circumstances, and associations available to the thinking part of the brain. Instantly the brain can determine if the pain is part of a minor irritating event and inconsequential, or it can ascertain that something is much more seriously wrong. Awareness of surroundings can be judged and consequences of reactions to the present pain can be gauged. For instance, a child is hurt when pushed down by a sibling. The reaction beyond that to the skinned knee itself can be greatly determined by the child's judgment of parental response. An athlete can be fouled in a soccer or hockey game and writhe on the ground a bit more dramatically if in the thinking part of the brain, the fourth circle of our model, he or she anticipates gaining a better call from the referee by doing so. Back pain that keeps one from working, from playing with the children, from engaging in intimacy with one's spouse, from joyfully anticipating the future is much more draining than back pain judged to be simple and short-lived. The experience of pain's effect on one's life is the primary determining factor of how one handles pain or painful situations. We all know that people can behave quite differently in similar circumstances.

When Does "Living with It" Start?

Does "living with it" start when "they" say that you have to live with it? So often patients have come to me after other doctors left them with that message. My own patients have said to me, "So, what you're telling me is that I'm going to have to live with this the rest of my life?" Or they'll couch it in terms of a contingency situation: "So, basically, Doc, if what you want to try doesn't work, I'll either have to get this big fusion surgery or I'll just have to live with it, right?"

Or they will have had a surgery, to heal lacerated nerves and tendons or to fix a spine problem or set a complex fracture, and they will be left with pain, numbness, weakness, clumsiness, or restricted motion. They survive a lifesaving brain surgery to remove a tumor or clip an aneurysm, but they are left with a significantly disfiguring paralysis of facial muscles and a palsied hand, difficulty speaking, and a poorly controllable eye. Then they are told, "You have to live with it . . . all of it." This is shocking news, and their first reaction is often one of despair: My God, my God, why have you forsaken me? *How* will I live with this?

My first response is always, "Well, the fact is, you *already are* 'living with it.' 'Living with it' does not start in some special time way out in the future, after you've done everything else. I do recognize, however, that you reach a specific point of coming to grips with 'living with it.'" Usually, we don't call into play the full force of our coping resources until we believe that all outside possibilities of correcting or alleviating the situation have been exhausted. When we truly begin to realize that we are about to be left on our own to deal with the problems at hand, when we are able to face facts and admit that for the foreseeable future we are not going to be rescued from our predicaments, we begin to call forth from within a new way of looking at our lives.

I also tell people that "forever" and the "rest of my life" are open canvasses of time, invention, discovery, and circumstance. For now, one might have to "live with" the limitations of what is available in pain medicines, therapy techniques, surgeries, and lifestyle changes. But there will always be new advances, new medicines, new options—things we cannot even imagine, some of which may apply to the problem at hand. We shall see in the Gospel stories ahead just how long many people had to wait for the miracle of Jesus to appear in their lives.

3

"CAN YOU RISK BEING ANGRY?"

The Tough Questions
You Have to Ask

As a patient in pain, you may experience real anger and frustration toward those close to you: the doctor to whom you are entrusting your care, who is sitting right in front of you, who is always late in clinic, leaving you waiting; your spouse, who is sitting next to you, who still thinks you should be helping more with the kids, or who may in subtle but devastating communications intimate that you are robbing him or her of dreams and plans and pleasures. And yes, these feelings certainly will be felt toward God.

It's one thing to get angry at a physical condition or an insurance provider. It is much more complex and risky to confront with anger your personal doctor, members of your family, or God. Each of these is too close, and none of them is going away. You have invested too much in these relationships to threaten them, even with legitimate problems and honest questions.

Your doctor, family member, and God have the power to hurt you, to "get back" at you for complaining or venting your anger at them. A trustworthy and seemingly competent doctor has the power to abandon you, to not really want to care for you anymore, to get tired of you. This doctor writes the prescriptions for your pain medication. This doctor may be the one writing your off-work or disability notes or handicap-parking slips. This doctor may be the only one willing to stick with you through this ordeal. It's no small thing to convey your frustration or dissatisfaction with him or her. Hence, you are caught in a situation of great vulnerability, because the doctor still hasn't cured you, gotten rid of all your pain, or at the very least guaranteed you through some letter that you will be financially secure forever. You are left with little choice but to live with the painful situation and with the doctor whom you depend upon to survive it. You are still the one desperately in need; therefore, you must control your anger.

Family interactions are even dicier. Whatever problem one member has, the others have in some way as well. In truth, family members will have to live with whatever you are living with, because they are living with you. Your family members may vent their frustrations at the doctor instead of at you. But once the doctors appointment is over, they must get back into the car with you, take the forty-five minute drive home, and then walk back into that home, in which there are few places to hide or get away from you or your pain and illness.

You as the patient may feel guilty for being dependent on your spouse or child to drive you to appointments, to therapies three times a week for months, to the drugstore constantly for new medicines or refills. They have to stand by you during those interminable, maddening hours in emergency rooms until someone finally gives you a pain shot at 3:00 a.m.—and for the fourth time this month. They sit in doctors' waiting rooms, and wait, and wait. Other hassles and obstacles abound, such as traffic and the inevitable mistakes of scheduling, the receptionist saying flatly, "I'm sorry, but I don't see your name on the list, and the doctor is completely booked today," or "The doctor was called out on an emergency and had to cancel."

On top of all this is the arguing with insurance companies, especially aggravating in those situations where you feel the continued need to prove the legitimacy of your disease or pain.

And what about this Being many of us call God, to whom we attribute all knowing, all power, all presence? Right now you are in pain and distress, and no rescue mission has been sent, no miracle has been delivered, no simple relief has even been experienced. Is it okay or even safe to complain to God about God?

Let's see: God is all-powerful and believed to be ultimately in control of life-and-death issues. If you express your anger to God about God, does the image of a bellowing, smoking, threatening Oz come to mind? Do you expect a lightning bolt to turn you into a charred smudge on the ground? Seriously, do you truly fear that God could make things worse or simply withdraw coldly from you and your insolence at not just accepting what has been sent from on high?

Rabbi Harold S. Kushner, in *When Bad Things Happen to Good People,* cites the example of a couple who lost a child and felt they were being punished by God for having been lax in their religious duties. Their fear of further punishment seemed to squelch their natural rage and pain at an inexplicable loss. "They sat there angry at God for having exacted his pound of flesh so strictly, but afraid to admit their anger for fear that he would punish them again. Life had hurt them, and religion could not comfort them. Religion was making them feel worse."

In a magnified way, complaining to God brings on the same types of fears as does complaining to your own doctor. Each has some form of power over you, perceived or real. This depends upon how you look at your caregivers, including your God, in relation to life's events and your own power, capacities, self-identity, and freedom to make choices and handle consequences.

Yet despite our best love and devotion to Jesus, human limitations leave us susceptible to the wearing nature of pain. We do not see the big picture, the brevity of life, the this-too-shall-pass philosophy because we are buried in pain, sadness, grief, loneliness, or despair. When a twenty-one-year-old athlete lies on a rotating hospital bed with no feeling or movement below his shoulders, having been told his spinal cord injury is likely permanent, there is no acceptance. There is total fear. One split second, one slip, one decision, one bizarre set of circumstances, and hell has swept over this young person's life like an inferno engulfing a pristine forest. What is destroyed will not grow back in our lifetime.

In *The Culture of Pain,* David B. Morris writes of a woman angry at what she must deal with after an injury:

> For Laura, what proved finally worse than the awful moment when the augur mangled her leg was a constant, irreparable pain that lingered long after the process of healing should have run its course. The leg in its healing had sealed in a tormenting and never-ending ache that gave her no freedom. She was in effect a prisoner shackled to her pain. She told me in a cold, emotionless tone that she wished the surgeons had simply cut off her leg at the knee. An artificial leg was something she could learn to live with: she could still cook, dance, work, take care of the kids. Chronic pain, however, had made the rest of her life a permanent daily torment.

What If People Question the Legitimacy of Your Pain?

More personal, hurtful, and insidiously difficult for patients and family members alike is the problem of legitimacy. Do you as the patient sense that your family really believes you? Do you as the family member really believe your loved one has all the pain and discomfort he or she claims? In these situations, love for the "loved one" is flattened and stretched to its tolerance limits. Why do none of the doctors seem able to find anything they can fix? A few may have provided explanations, but some of the doctors and therapists say they're puzzled as to why this situation is so problematic. Most other patients do so much better by now. Doubt creeps in, both for you as patient and for you as family. The patient starts to feel self-conscious about his or her lack of credibility. The family starts to wonder what is really going on—dare they ask, "Could this be something psychological, Doctor? Is this what people call 'psychosomatic'?"

Remember, pain is invisible. It is personal. It is hard to quantify, and it is hard to compare. Telling yourself that there must be others with much worse pain and more serious conditions; reminding yourself of the starving millions around the world or those who have undergone torture—these psychological tactics really do nothing to alleviate your personal moment of pain. Your brain's pain centers couldn't care less for games of relativity right now. You admit that you're losing the battle to will away the pain, but even such an admission does not gain you rescue. The pain bores in, throbs, squeezes, burns, shoots, stabs. And others around you may begin to get tired of hearing about it, especially when the doctors have run out of options.

But there are times when it's entirely appropriate to ask the tough questions. Sean would practically seethe every time I brought up the idea of getting him back into some type of modified duty at work. He was a carpenter and had hurt his shoulder, wrist, back, and knee falling off a high ladder while working on a construction project. It boiled down to the fact that he couldn't stand his boss and blamed him for almost all the problems he was going through.

I asked him how his boss had caused him to fall. Had he misaligned the ladder? Was he not holding on as the spotter, or did he leave a rung broken? Did he force Sean into a dangerous job? Sean admitted that his boss hadn't even been on the site.

"Really?" I said. "So your boss didn't actually push you off the ladder and cause you to fall and get hurt?"

"No, I was there on my own."

"Well, the reason I ask it that way is that the anger you have about this injury and all your pain seems to be always directed at your boss. Like it was his fault. Here all this time I thought you were mad at him for the fact that you got hurt in the first place because of something he had done. At least that's the way it all comes across."

"I'm just ticked at him because he's been such an SOB about the insurance payments and my back pay."

"Do you think that has anything to do with the fact that you're always telling me you're not ready to go back to work? You know, you've had the best treatment with the best physical and occupational therapists I know. Nothing is broken or torn. You should be fine, but you're miserable. You're angry, Sean; perhaps rightly so. But you're no longer hurt."

Cultural Factors That Influence Your Pain

A given culture will display some common collective behavior patterns in response to pain. Some Asian cultures are incredibly stoic in the face of what peoples of other cultures may consider near torture-level pain. Some Pacific Island and African cultures ritualize the tolerance of pain through degrees of body piercing or rites of passage that most Western cultures would consider extreme and unapproachable. Other cultures seem to have reinforced opposite behaviors. Southern European (Spanish, Portuguese, Italian, Greek), Latin American, African American, Arab, and Jewish peoples all can be very demonstrative and expressive in comparison with some of the Asian and northern European peoples.

Do people of these different cultures experience the same physical pain? Is there, in fact, the presence of the same amount of tissue damage, the same wiring of nerve signals and registration of biological pain in the thalamic regions of their brains? Do they all have, in a sense, the same first, second, and third circles of the pain diagram described earlier? If so, there must be tremendous suppressive power of the associative centers, adding up lifetimes of observed, learned, and acted-out responses in the fourth circle, in order to manifest the stoicism often demonstrated.

What is the mechanism of stoicism? Is it a mere matter of the will? Is it the personality of a culture planted in the psyches of individuals who are indoctrinated by that culture throughout their lives? And is it possible that, over a lifetime of such behaviors, the internal physiology of the body and the brain is altered? What if this learning has been selected out genetically over generations so that biology reinforces culture and behavior, and vice versa? In some religious body-piercing rituals, there seems to be this overlap of mental pain tolerance and physiologic adjustment, wherein multiple objects pierced through skin and tissue produce no bleeding and seemingly no outward sign of pain.

The point is that individuals can handle and manage their pains and sufferings in different fashions because of the powerful influences of the larger entity we call culture. We must all be attuned to the fact that there can exist dramatically different responses to what may be very similar diseases, procedures, or situations. We must also be aware of our own perspectives, not presuming our viewpoints to be some gold standard for all peoples of the earth, many of whom may have been taught behaviors quite distinct from our own.

Can You Be Honest with Yourself?

In psychosocial dynamics there does exist what in medicine is called "secondary gain." Medical professionals can become suspicious when they are unable to find answers within the bounds of their trusted techniques and textbooks and tests. What might a patient, or even a family, be getting out of the situation continuing as it is? Obvious secondary-gain benefits may in fact be present, to a degree, in work- or personal-injury cases, where substantial sums of money are at stake. The worse off you appear and the longer you appear that way, the more money you "win." You may never have to work again. You may really get to "make the bastards pay." On the other hand, you may just be following the advice of your attorney, in fear that if you don't, you won't get anything at all or the firm will drop your case. At this stage, you are too deep into it, financially and emotionally, to back off now. You have been out of work or been laid off. Perhaps even the company you worked for has folded. Meanwhile, time drags on and bills pile up and animosity grows. Secondary gain can be a very sharp two-edged sword.

Other secondary gains are more difficult to discern and to admit. Let's say you're an accountant with migraines and neck pain, and you really hate your job or your boss. In your eyes, there is no way out of the job situation through further education or through quitting and looking for something more satisfying. You've been off work several times due to incapacitating pain, and now you have a medical condition on your record. Your employer is getting tired of your unreliability. Who else would hire you now? Certainly you won't be able to make the same kind of money by doing lots of overtime like you used to. If you have to break into another line of work, how do you get qualified without spending time and money on education; how do you get by on the low wages of an entry-level position? And who in this day and age is going to cover you with medical benefits if you have a "preexisting condition"? The only way out of pain and a painful situation is to remain ill and apply for disability. The reverse secondary gain in these circumstances is that you cannot afford to get better. Doing so seems to leave you in a worse, more precarious, uncertain financial position. This is a very real concern for many individuals recovering from injury. Judging true pain compared to the pain stemming from anxiety is difficult. There are legitimate risks to healing. Such issues are addressed in the specific discussions of some of the Gospel healings elsewhere in this book.

What of secondary gain within the intimacy of your home? When roles within the family change because of illness, the very personal dynamics among family members change, as well. A spouse has to be taken care of when he or she was previously always called upon to be the stronger one. A parent gets to hold on to a teenage or adult child by playing the caretaker role. A parent gets to stay in touch with children and grandchildren by being in need of frequent help, visits, or transportation. Sexuality between spouses can be avoided, if that is the goal, by using pain or risk of injury as an excuse. Household chores or parental tasks can be avoided or shirked if the real or perceived risk of pain is employed as a negotiating tool. Pain as a threat or as a weapon can be incredibly powerful. On the other hand, we as family caregivers can withdraw, be less sympathetic, turn accusatory and disbelieving, never be around, or go on making plans and enjoying the pleasures of life without involving the suffering patient. Plain and simple, we can get tired of it all.

Doctors, nurses, therapists, and families must be wary, however, of doubting the underlying presence of true pain, suffering, and illness in patients and relatives, no matter how poorly or suspiciously they may be behaving in our eyes. Statistically, there are very few patients who are totally faking pain. Circumstances may lead patients to "symptom-magnify," as we doctors like to term this behavior. It is difficult to convey to another how much one is suffering. Thus, some patients may exaggerate postures or groans or helplessness in attempts to "show" their pain, especially when all the fancy tests don't show anything "objective" to justify their "subjective" pain. In the end, most would rather be completely pain free and leading normal lives outside doctors' offices and pharmacies. Some people do seek to compensate the lack of love and care in their daily lives with the attention of doctors, nurses, and therapists. Most, however, would rather fill this void at home.

When medical science cannot explain the symptoms, the challenge is often put back on the patient to explain the illness. There may in fact exist some secondary gain as described above, but healthcare professionals and family members must resist the urge to blame the patient or imply that he or she is faking or simply hysterical. In *The Culture of Pain,* David B. Morris writes:

Pain ranks prominently among the most familiar symptoms of hysteria. . . . The hysterical woman seemed a labyrinth of curious and largely unresponsive pains. . . . The hysterical patient lived in a world where pain flowed continuously through her body and settled in the most unexpected places. . . . Doctors did not need to wait for a full theory of psychoanalysis before suspecting that the often diffuse, confusing, multiple symptoms of hysteria originated mainly in the patient's mind. Women were regularly suspected of faking illness. . . . Hysteria quickly became medical code for made-up, factitious, or imaginary illness. . . . At issue was the question of whether a woman's pain was real. . . . The positivist medicine that emerged in the nineteenth century, however, rejected the traditional view that pain was an emotion. Doctors increasingly identified pain with organic lesions of the nervous system. A nineteenth-century woman who complained of pains incompatible with current medical knowledge about the nervous system thus ran the serious risk of finding her illness dismissed as imaginary. The hysteric in effect became the victim of a double affliction. She suffered not only from multiple pains but also from the suspicion of male doctors that her pain was merely the gossamer product of an overheated, labile, sexually deranged, morally corrupt female imagination. Further, it was commonly thought that women did not so much imagine their pain as deliberately fake it, and such suspicions have proved hard to dislodge.

Christ looked beyond symptoms in his interactions with people and their disorders. Whatever the factors contributing to an individual's illness or crippling ailment, he saw first a suffering creature. He recognized the interplay of physical, emotional, social, and spiritual suffering. While a person suffering pain must wrestle with how to cope with it and even how to communicate about it, that person's caregivers, professional or family, must get beyond their personal (albeit human) reactions to, and judgments of, other people's pain complaints and pain behaviors. The real task for everyone involved is to assess the best course of action.

When we, as suffering patients, encounter doubt in those we love and need the most, it will help our own minds if we accept that this is natural and common. Such disbelief hurts, to be sure, especially on top of all the pains we already endure. Yet we must in our hearts pray to remain patient with our caregivers and with our loved ones. And there is no limit to the help we can ask of our God.

How Far Will You Go for a Cure?

Many of our scientific discoveries can be called miraculous. We almost don't see them as such any longer. We can grow impatient for the instant cures. And we can run up against some tough choices, even morally, when we are desperate to relieve pain or save our lives. The system for organ transplants seeks to protect us from the corruption or unfairness such desperation can bring. Stem-cell research is another mixed blessing. Stem cells are thought to have the capacity to be scientifically engineered or programmed to form specific tissues or to produce needed body chemicals such as hormones, antibodies, or neurotransmitters. The problem is that stem cells can be obtained from aborted embryos, and embryos used for donor stem cells will then be aborted. An interpretation of such is that humanity creates and harvests one set of lives to "feed" and sustain another. For what or for whom would we cross that line?

It is as if the devil is taking us up to the top of our own towers of temptation, showing us our futures: In the face of terminal pancreatic cancer, would we like the option of a new pancreas? Lying paralyzed for life with a spinal cord injury, would we like new, functioning nerve cells implanted that would allow us to walk and function normally again? If our child had acute leukemia, would we like an instant, easily transfusable, exact-match replacement blood supply for him or her, to avoid the suffering of long, painful treatments that could still fail? Your leg, amputated as a result of diabetes, a tumor, or a trauma could be replaced with a new one. You could cure your ulcerative colitis or Crohn's disease with a new, perfectly functioning colon. Your hemorrhaging uterus could be exchanged for a new one. Your Parkinson's diseased brain could be replenished to its natural dopamine balance, allowing you to move and talk fluidly again. Your depression or bipolar disease could be eliminated by resupplying the needed neurotransmitters.

All the glistening jewels of a normal, whole, healthy, functioning body would be laid before us, if we but chose to take this one uncomfortable step of allowing the scientists, doctors, and researchers to use leftover embryos. They're going to die anyway. They could be harvested for the good of humankind. Or would you prefer to remain blind or paralyzed because of your high morals? It's easy to talk about religious ethics until our own lives and sacrifices are on the line.

One young couple left the fertility clinic hopeful, yet somewhat troubled. Devoutly Catholic, they realized they would have to weigh the odds of conceiving a life through in vitro fertilization versus conceiving too many and as a result having to abort the "extras." The more eggs they donated, the better their chances that at least one would become fertilized. And the more eggs successfully fertilized and then implanted in the uterus, the higher the odds that at least one of them would "take" and develop into a full, successful pregnancy, and a child of their own. But if multiple eggs were fertilized, the young woman couldn't have them all implanted, for what if they all survived? It would become a complicated multiple pregnancy. The doctors had no such concerns. Their technology allowed them to easily freeze or get rid of the "excess" fertilized eggs, and to abort the "extra" pregnancies if too many embryos implanted. Their goal was the successful pregnancy of one. The strategy was just to increase the odds. Discarding the rest was a minor cost of success.

The couple, however, chose to always opt for lower numbers in their efforts. They would donate only the number of eggs they thought safe to implant if all were successfully fertilized, which meant three at the most for any one cycle of in vitro attempt. This lowered their chances for success, but in their hearts they could make no other choice. After many rounds, they were unsuccessful. Deciding to stop the effort was a truly sad moment. Yet after the long ordeal of laboring to become pregnant, the couple was blessed with several children through adoption. Life was given to them through a different portal, but the mystery and the joy and the love were there all the same. God granted the miracle in spite of the pain. Other couples may face the challenging choices differently; the struggles and the anguish are no less difficult, no matter the outcomes. The goal is good. The path is hard.

Let us move on now to the main mission of the book: the exploration of the miracles in the Gospels. As with this young couple, how true it is that the miracle, the healing, comes in spite of the pain. Too often we look at miracles as relieving all pain and suffering, all maladies and illnesses. Seemingly simple in their moments of blessing and transformation, Christ's cures were surely not so simple within the contexts of the lives in which they occurred, lives very much like our own.

The Stories to Come

The stories and experiences of people and patients today are not really any different from those of people throughout history. In particular, the individuals we read about in the Gospels are very much like us. I think that too often we look upon them as distant, specially chosen lottery winners in ancient robes with strange diseases of leprosy, blindness, or demonic possession. We may not take their healings as factual experiences of real people to whom we can relate. I see them as archetypes of the patients I see in practice every day, of the sad tales of friends and their families, or of strangers on the news each night.

If we look more closely behind the scenes of the miracles, and more creatively at the lives involved compared to our own, perhaps we can understand the parallels therein. In so doing, maybe we can then see more clearly that the God whose power transformed lives in Matthew, Mark, Luke, and John is just as available and powerful in our lives. We tend to think that if we had been there, we of course would have put all our faith in Jesus. Why do we look at our lives at this very moment any differently? It is not that we don't sincerely pray. I just wonder if we allow ourselves the gift of the answers, the same answers given to so many in the Gospels when they encountered the healing love of Jesus.

The following chapters bring together the Gospel stories and our stories. Churchgoers hear this done in homilies and sermons week after week. As a doctor dealing with people in pain, I hope I bring a different angle to some of these familiar passages. Even if you don't agree with my particular interpretation of a Gospel message, or you can't relate to the patient I present, I ask that you pray for something else in your own heart to be stirred, or even jarred. We all do this, I'm sure, when on a given day we find ourselves tired and trying to follow what we consider an uninspiring service. God can obviously reach us beyond the limits of any speaker or author, in particular beyond those of this author. If you've read this far, your heart and mind are already open and searching for that which is beyond the print on this paper.

In most of the following chapters, contemporary patient stories are juxtaposed with Gospel patient stories. I include a reflection prayer at the end of some of these chapters, trying to give voice to the feelings within that relate to the message of our Lord's own actions and words. I then present brief sets of applied life questions to bridge the spiritual to the practical. The book is not a novel, and thus one chapter does not have to be read before another in any particular order. I will say that the ending chapters have to do more with the heavier topics of death, dying, and suffering in general. I pray that you are encouraged and strengthened by the journey, and that the words bring you some solace, wisdom, and inspiration, however they are meant to, as the Holy Spirit imparts God's graces to you. Come, then. Let us meet some of these people, and ourselves, too.

4

"IF YOU WANT TO, YOU CAN MAKE ME WELL."*

The Anatomy of a Miracle

There is a very short, simple passage titled in some translations "A Leper" or "Cure of a Leper" presented in the Gospels of Matthew (8:1–4), Mark (1:40–45), and Luke (5:12–16). With no great fanfare, a man came forward. For some reason, the Gospel writers chose to memorialize this man, among the thousands who received cures. Though he appeared early in Mark's Gospel, many others had been cured already by this time. Even so, this man seems to have been one of the first to recognize the healing power present in Jesus, for it was this man's proclamations of his miracle story that made it "impossible for Jesus to enter a town openly" (Mark 1:45).

A Suffering Man Takes a Risk

The leper steps out, and thus he stands out. He risks himself merely by identifying himself before Jesus. We don't know how long it's

---

* Some chapter titles are paraphrases and not direct quotes from the Bible.

taken him to get up enough courage to do this. We don't know if he's hesitated before at other opportunities he may have had. Maybe he's come to Jesus on his own, after the crowds have gone, because he fears creating distress by bringing his horrible disease close to the other sick people and their families. He may be educated and wise in many ways, through his own quiet, lonely striving. For all we know, he might have been a high-level official or business-man before contracting his leprosy. Whatever the circumstances, he engages others with respect and deference.

He does not waste Jesus' or anyone else's time. He doesn't beat around the bush with a long story of his woes. He says simply, "If you wish, you can make me clean" (Luke 5:12). He believes a miracle is possible, but he does not demand it. It is more that he trusts in the power of Jesus, rather than speaking from a place of entitlement, insisting that he be rid of his problem.

This leper risks presenting his desire to the person whom he believes to be the source that can fulfill it. The man lays his life before Jesus, trusting the goodness he believes to exist in him. The healing gift is shared by the two of them, and each grows in the process. Do not doubt this in your own healing interactions. *Each participant is partner in giving over the self to the moment of transformation.* Thus, as much as this leper is asking to be cured, he is also calling forth a response from the healer. This man's very actions and initiative serve to elicit from Jesus the power and goodness existing in him.

Jesus and the leper connect without delaying, analyzing, or cal-culating. Christ does not stop to weigh the physical and social risks of interacting with this outcast and his disease. He doesn't turn the man away, complaining that he should have come earlier when everyone else was there, that he is through for the day, or that he is tired.

Jesus meets this man right where he is, matching the man's directness with his own immediate response. There are no lines in the Gospels that separate the leper's statement, "If you wish, you can make me clean," from Jesus' response. Jesus stretched out his hand

and touched him and said, "I will do it. Be made clean" (Matthew 8:2–3). We can imagine their eyes meeting and all being said in that exchange of gazes. In an instant, they have touched each other at the core. So incredible and powerful to imagine, isn't it? Do we ever sense this to be possible in our own lives?

"Lord, I am not worthy to receive you. Only say the word, and I will be healed."

Catholics say these words in every Mass just before receiving Communion. According to the Catholic faith, we can enter into a church every single day of our lives, attend Mass, and walk up to Jesus himself, with all our troubles, just as the people in the Gospel stories, and say to him, "Lord, if you will it, you can heal me." Do we know what we are really saying with these words? Are we truly focused at that moment, enough to realize that we are repeating the very words spoken by the lepers and the blind in the Gospels who were fully open to the power of Christ to heal them?

When we bring true faith to such a moment, as did the leper, and when we trust in God's knowledge of what is best for us and of what is really our deepest desire, we can hear God say, "It is your faith that has been your salvation." That faith accepts that somehow our lives have been changed, blessed, healed. How deeply do we believe the words we speak? As with so many prayers repeated out of habit, how many times do these crucial words slip from our mouths empty, powerless to produce the miracles for which we so desperately long?

The leper did not demand of our Lord. He expressed complete, doubtless faith—faith that Jesus had the power to heal the illness presented. His faith rested in the acknowledgment and acceptance ahead of time of the "if you will it." We each come before Jesus with the same opportunity that the leper had.

The leper teaches us to act out of courage and decisiveness, to come directly to moments of change. This man shows us how to bring our broken bodies to God with a readiness to move on, to get going with our lives. What if Christ had instead said to him, "Come follow me," or "Go fetch a donkey that your Master may ride into Jerusalem"? Are we prepared to come to God in our prayers for miracles with an openness to hear whatever God has to offer us?

Jesus Responds with Uplifting Pity

Jesus was "moved with pity" when the man knelt before him (Mark 1:41). In the Gospels, this pity that Jesus often displays seems an indication of his profound love and sensitivity to the suffering of the people he encounters.

Our own pity for others often carries with it a need to distance ourselves—we want to draw away from the pathetic sight before us. Almost reflexively we keep ourselves safe—from "catching" the paralysis of the person in the wheelchair, the blindness of the person with the cane and glasses standing next to us near the curb, the craziness of the man talking to himself, the poverty of the disheveled woman asking for money. We are usually afraid of contacting or feeling the suffering around us too intimately, fearful of being sucked into it. It may grab us and demand something. It may create too much of a scene. We are embarrassed. We are too self-conscious, not wanting our routines disturbed or our anonymity disrupted. We may even attempt to suppress the desires of others in order to protect our own comfort zones, as did the crowds who scolded the blind Bartimaeus, "telling him to be silent" (Mark 10:48).

When Jesus shows pity, he always comes *closer* to those in need of him, touching and uplifting them. No matter what "leprosy" we carry, we can know that God will not back away from us in disgust, even if that is how we ourselves might react or how we experience others reacting to us. He will not distance himself from us because of our "badness." He will not bypass us on his way to somewhere or someone more important or safe.

Hearing the Message in the Healing

In Mark 2 and Luke 5, the story of the paralytic at Capernaum tells of large crowds surrounding Jesus so that many feared they would not get in to see him. Four men who carried a paralyzed man on his mat were not to be deterred from completing their mission. They actually climbed up onto the dwelling, made a hole in the roof over Jesus, and lowered the man down in front of him. A bold move, to say the least. The question is not whether this man was in any greater need of Jesus' attention, or whether he was more worthy or his friends more devout than anyone else waiting to see the Master. Who knows if the man on the mat himself was resisting the "pushiness" of the four men who carried him? Perhaps he didn't even want to be there. It is obvious, however, that these four men felt the need to present their friend to Jesus for healing.

We may or may not recognize the more serious illnesses we carry with us to God, or to our doctors. The first thing Jesus said to the man lowered down to him, in front of everyone gathered there, was, "Your sins are forgiven." Do you think that was what the man or his four friends were expecting to be greeted with after having gone through all those dramatic motions? Jesus is our Creator and knows more than we know about what we need. He speaks to us for all time when he says, "Your sins are forgiven. *Now,* you can stand up and walk and be healed through and through." Though we may constantly cry to God to be relieved of some malady or problem, he may want us to look first into what more seriously ails us. When we feel that God is not hearing us, we might check to see if we are hearing God.

This story also shows us the communal nature of miracles and healing. When we are too beaten down to even try to help ourselves, we pray for those who can find it in their hearts to help us. Those with addiction problems are a special challenge to friends and family. The problem is often not recognized as such by the person afflicted.

It demands a great deal of energy and commitment on the part of those concerned to stay the course in these trying situations. The true miracle in an addicted person's life is that God keeps inspiring others to enter the fray with help. Illness, pain, and suffering are rarely isolated conditions, and we all need the love and support of our communities to manifest God's love to us tangibly. With this in mind, remember to go out of your own way for the person alone and in need. God walks, talks, touches, and heals through one of us. You are on call. Be alert. The miracle may be in you.

The Gospels Speak Today, Too

As we look back on the miracle stories in the Gospels, will we be able to transpose what we learn from Jesus' actions two thousand years ago to our present struggles with pain, illness, loss, and disappointment? While in the midst of our real experiences of chronic headaches or back pain, nausea or fatigue from cancer therapies, paralysis from strokes or spinal cord injuries, and so on, does it mean anything to us that Jesus cured a man of his leprosy? Do parents gain hope for their daughter's health because they read of Jesus restoring health to a little girl who was thought dead? When you receive the news that you have pancreatic cancer, AIDS, or ALS, does the story of Jesus raising Lazarus inspire any hope of a reprieve from your perceived medical death sentence?

For most individuals described in the Gospels, the first step is in some way the acknowledgment or awareness of the need for healing. Life is out of order. This can pertain to a very concrete and obvious physical disease or dysfunction, or it can pertain to the more insidious aspects of an unhealthy lifestyle.

As we have already seen in the story of the leper, many courageous people in the Gospels stepped out of the crowd to call to Jesus, even when others, embarrassed or irritated, tried to quiet them. These people took the initiative. They took risks. They were often in a process of searching. They humbled themselves, asked for help, and expected miracles.

How often do we chide each other, seriously or not, with the caution, "But don't expect miracles"? Are we open to what miracles may actually look like in our lives, or are we limiting our vision to what we have always thought miracles *should* look like? Perhaps we suffer or doubt much of the time because we do not see the actions of God that are already occurring before us, so sure are we of what is supposed to happen if God were really present and listening to our cries. Can we move from what we perceive to be our urgent needs to an awareness of the deeper relief and cure available to us through God?

Sometimes we allow that a "guardian angel" may have crossed our paths and provided the small reprieve or the gentle word we needed. But we don't often label these Divine gestures as true miracles. We still wait for the big flashes, the total relief, the complete disappearance of all that ails us.

Understandably, we may be begging and waiting for the waking to full health of a child in a coma. Sincerely, we may offer our desires each day for God to have the cancer eradicated by the medicines, the coronary arteries opened by the surgery, the seizures finally stop plaguing a spouse. These are the big, actual miracles for which we say the deepest of prayers, though we are certainly grateful to the angels for the smaller cups of water passed to us along the course of our marathons.

We can never know the moment when our miracles will be made manifest to us. Life is a blend of living with what we have been given and searching for more, for ourselves or for others. How we search and how we live may be part of the healing in the first place. If we are granted a defining instant of change or revelation, it is God's gift to grant and our responsibility to recognize and to grow as a result. But it is often the ordinariness of the events and opportunities that deceive us into looking past them for something more.

This was perhaps the failing of so many who missed God in Christ because they had been looking for something grander. Others, though, were able to see goodness so near to them. By responding, they opened the door to greater possibilities. They came as they were, and accepted and received healing as it was offered.

Too often, when patients don't hear what they want to hear, they leave available healing on the table, because it doesn't add up to enough for them. It's too little result for too much bother. It's merely another medicine, or another technique, another appointment they'll have to make. I just saw a man who listened to my evaluation of his MRI scan and my plan to systematically try to locate his primary source of pain. He heard only that all his pain wouldn't go away in one shot.

Many who suffer often don't recognize that the next cup of water may get them just far enough to reach the finish line. Sometimes bigger things don't happen because people don't bring their full selves into the encounter in the first place. They come with only the dregs of their impatience and the neediness to be done with it all. They fear another disappointment and therefore can't see the potential in the partial solutions. Whether the decision is to stop smoking, stop drinking alcohol, stop taking drugs, lose weight, deal with pain, or live in spite of illness or life's disappointments, miracles occur because we finally bring ourselves in courageous integrity to single, specific points of change.

The Power of Prayer

Beyond psychic energy and forces, what about the power of prayer? Can prayer be tested? Dr. Larry Dossey wrote two books on the subject: *Healing Words: The Power of Prayer and the Practice of Medicine* and *Prayer Is Good Medicine: How to Reap the Healing Benefits of Prayer.* He explores the scientific side of spirituality. He concludes that "in its simplest form, prayer is an attitude of the heart—a matter of being, not doing." It is a "desire to contact the Absolute, however it may be conceived." One of the most effective forms of prayer, discerned through the multiple studies reviewed and the conclusions of their various authors, is the "Thy will be done" prayer. Dossey states in *Healing Words*:

> There may be important spiritual lessons here. Because prayer can violate the categories of past, present, and future, it seems timeless. Thus one of its functions may be to awaken us to the "eternal now," the experience of timelessness described by the mystics of every esoteric religious tradition. Perhaps this is one of the lessons inherent in one of the most universal of prayers, "Thy will be done." Divisions in time are absent from this prayer: it does not say, "Thy will be done today or tomorrow." "Be" implies the infinitude in time that always has been ascribed to the Almighty. "Thy will be done" denotes an eternal pervasiveness of the divine will. Perhaps the prayer "Thy will be done" can awaken us to a new way of judging time and a new way of thinking about the role of prayer in health.

This prayer acknowledges our limited awareness of what is truly right for us, for our loved ones, or for the world in the overwhelming complexities of life and its inherent conflicts. It acknowledges our powerlessness, our need for help, and our belief in the mystery of the benevolence and power of the being we call God. It relieves us of guilt and burdens, and provides us with a calm sense of giving over that which we cannot control. It does not imply passive inaction. It does not imply easiness. A friend pointed out to me how she felt when she was praying for her seriously ill mother: "Lord, I'll pray 'Thy will be done,' but not if your will is that my mother dies. I cannot pray for that. I just can't."

Dossey writes, "We need to recall at these times that prayer, in its function as a bridge to the Absolute, has no failure rate. It works one hundred percent of the time—unless we prevent this realization by remaining oblivious to it." Bridget Meehan, in *The Healing Power of Prayer*, adds, "The struggle and pain endured in this life need not destroy our faith in the reality of God's presence." God understands us in those moments. It is we who as yet do not understand God at those moments. That's all right. He promises we will one day.

A Review of Gospel Principles about Healing

Change often comes first when we acknowledge and stay aware of our brokenness and need for healing. We mix humility with trust in a power greater than the self. This power is absolutely good and absolutely free to exercise itself on our behalf. Common to all the healing stories is Jesus' deep compassion for people in their suffering, his desire to lift them up out of their pain, and his assurance that God is tireless in his mercy toward people.

The petitioners in the Gospels do not believe that they are *owed* the gift of healing. Nonetheless, as children, they sometimes place themselves unabashedly before the power of God in full expectation, trusting in the love of a wise, benevolent father. At other times, they must first of all overcome the fear, guilt, and weakness that hinder them. Often the miracles occur only after much effort, perseverance, and searching. Risk, courage, and valor play their parts in the process of change.

The healing experience is active, not passive. Someone—the healer, the sick, or members of the community—needs to do something in order to effect the transformation. We are inspired to search out God with our needs, while God ever seeks to be found. In the process, we may be called to change or to carry on, even when we do not fully understand the present moment.

Miracles may require a little ritual. They may require the help of others. They ask much of our faith and our trust, especially when we don't understand why we must endure the time and pain they often require. In the end, there remains the mystery of suffering and the very need for what we call miracles. We sometimes think of miracles in the Gospel stories and in our various faith traditions as simply enigmatic, spectacular, isolated events in world history. We identify them as rare, unexplainable, dramatic, and unexpected—even if prayed for—moments of Divine intervention, generally having taken place in the past. For many of the faithful, however, they are not so rare at all.

When the paralytic first heard that his sins were forgiven, was his heart receptive to a different kind of miracle than the one he had been seeking? Is there faith enough in God's love, wisdom, and power to trust that whatever happens in response to our prayers, we in fact truly receive all that we pray for? And do we pray with enough faith to risk naming that which our hearts genuinely desire, while at the same time acknowledging humbly that, in the midst of our pains and confusion, we sometimes just don't know what that is? Thus we say to the Lord, I know that if you will it, you can heal me of whatever it is in me that most needs healing; and I trust that in your goodness, you will grant me what is best for me, though I may not be able to recognize it right now.

5

"DAUGHTER, YOUR FAITH HAS CURED YOU."

The Effort That Healing Requires

Within the intimacy of a doctor's office, many profound things can occur. Despite the rushed and pressured atmosphere of today's managed care system, the personal and private moments between doctors and patients can still produce some sacred space. Yet there really is a sense that available time is too compressed for anything sacred to occur. Waiting rooms are full of frustrated patients and families, irritated at how long they have been sitting, at how far behind the doctor is, at how long it's taking the surgeon to get back from the "emergency" at the hospital.

The mantra of the fed-up patient is the cliché "My time is as important as the doctor's! I'll start charging him for the time I'm wasting here when I have other things to do!" My response has often been to say that it is not my time that is being traded off for theirs, but that of all the other patients being seen that day. The patients later in the day will have to complain to the patients earlier in the day as to why they took up so much of the doctor's time. Most doctors are no longer out playing golf somewhere, trust me. They are running around trying to catch up. It is difficult to balance the time it takes to handle people, their illnesses, and their concerns. Our society demands instant service and solutions, yet complains that doctors never spend enough time listening to patients' problems and answering their questions.

Those Who Suffer Must Also Seek

Whether illnesses are seriously life threatening, such as cancer or heart disease or strokes, or whether they relate more to pain and dysfunction, the person bearing the suffering is anxious to be seen. We all want our problems addressed quickly, our worst fears allayed, our treatments begun, our pains alleviated, and our lives back on track. Yet we don't want to be rushed when it is our turn to see the doctor, even when he or she is struggling to stay on schedule. We need time to explain ourselves, and we want time to have our disorders explained to us. So, do we wait six weeks to see the doctor who only schedules a limited number of patients each day, or do we go today and wait three hours in the reception area as an "add-on," while the ten patients ahead of us keep asking questions? Tough choices for all involved.

And often, the better the physician we are trying to see, the harder it is to get an appointment with him or her. This leads to frustration and fear. We don't know how serious our symptoms are. We don't know what they portend for us. At times, we dread the lurking threat of cancer, spreading through our bodies before we can get in to see the doctor, obtain all the necessary tests, and formulate a plan. As in any situation where we have very little power or knowledge and yet very great need, we feel vulnerable and perhaps resentful at our dependence on the services of others.

It is hard to bite your tongue when the doctor finally walks into your little exam room after you've been sitting there for forty-five minutes, on top of the thirty minutes you spent in the reception area bored with old magazines, wondering whether to cancel an afternoon meeting or to just leave because you have to pick up your kids from school or day care. But you need this doctor right now, and you want him or her totally invested in solving your particular problem. It can be a tough first couple of minutes as you try to suppress the steam rising within you. So you politely ask your questions and try to refocus on why you're here in the first place.

From the doctor's perspective, it can seem like one is behind as soon as the morning alarm goes off. The rest of the day is a continuous run: trying to remain calm with patients, listening to them carefully to figure out what's really going on, writing down answers to phone messages that keep popping up on clipboards, all the while worrying a little about being sued for God knows what.

There is many a night, arriving home at nine or ten o'clock or awakened by a page at three in the morning, when I feel too tired from this job. I wonder whether I'm exhausted because I'm not getting enough out of my work, not putting enough into my work, or maybe just leaving too much of myself in my work. A friend advised me to discern the difference between the physical and mental tiredness that comes from putting forth a good effort, and the draining of one's spirit from struggling where one shouldn't be struggling.

How did Christ manage when the throngs came out to be touched, healed, cured? We know that at the end of the day, he, too, was tired, that he was probably exhausted physically, emotionally, and spiritually. He had to retreat to the quiet of his boat and get out among the refreshing sea breezes of the open waters. He would retreat to the desert to rejuvenate and replenish his own being in the solitude. Sometimes he would choose to be in the company of his small group of friends for support, while at other times he would send them off and slip away on his own.

Healing does, in fact, take effort. It took the expenditure of the power within Jesus, both physical and mental. And it took effort on the part of the person being healed.

Our Desire to "Fix It"

We in Western civilization, and particularly in the United States, have come to identify health as a freedom from disease, pain, discomfort, inconvenience, and stress. If any of these interrupt our busy lives, we seek from the medical industry quick evaluations, answers, and corrections so that we can get on with our "normalcy." Of course, only those privileged with "normal" lives in the first place have the luxury of saying this. Still, as a culture and society, we face disorder with an eagerness to eliminate it.

In our personal lives, we treat disease somewhat the same way as the military approaches war. We seek the latest smart bomb that can surgically strike at the bad guys within us while not harming the good guys. We want it done as quickly and cleanly and inexpensively as possible. We want no occupying forces remaining within us. We want no mess. We look to modern, highly technological medicine to come up with miracle drugs and minimalist procedures in order to get the job done. And why not?

At the same time, we hear a rising lament about the sterility of scientific medicine. We complain about the lack of personal attention we receive in running from one specialist to another. Finally, we are just tired of it all. "I want this to just go away." Isn't it amazing how much it can hurt to have to work and persevere in order to get rid of one's pain, in order to persist in the search for one's miracle?

Healing Power Had Gone out from Him

One of the most well-known Gospel healing stories tells of a woman who seems to "steal" power from Jesus by touching the hem of his cloak. She is the woman with a hemorrhage of twelve years' duration. Her condition is described as incurable. From Mark's version, we know she has been searching desperately for help: "She had suffered greatly at the hands of many doctors and had spent all she had. Yet she was not helped but only grew worse" (Mark 5:26). Can anyone identify with her?

Isn't it amazing how real this part of the story is? We sometimes think of the miracle stories as so glorified and otherworldly that we cannot relate to them or to the people in them who had leprosy, who were blind beggars at a roadside, or who were possessed of evil spirits. Yet how much more connected with this woman can a contemporary patient, who has a long history of illness and is searching for medical attention, be? She has gone from doctor to doctor, exhausting her savings, has been deemed incurable, and has only become worse for all the treatments she has undergone. This woman could be you.

No other details are provided, as the story moves immediately to the point where she comes up behind Jesus in the crowd. Before we get to that, though, let's think a little of her situation and how she may have arrived at this point. Who knows how weak and exhausted she was with chronic, fatiguing anemia from her long history of blood loss. Who knows if she felt faint and dizzy every time she stood up, which significant anemia will cause. How much effort did it take for her to do anything, becoming short of breath with even the slightest activity because her low blood count limited the oxygen available in her circulation?

How far did she have to walk to find Jesus? How many times had she tried? How many stairs did she have to climb? How much fighting through the throngs to even get near Jesus? Remember, "as he went, the crowds almost crushed him" (Luke 8:42)—so, too, they must have almost crushed her as she was jostled and bumped in her mission to get close enough to touch him. With her platelet count low from all the years of hemorrhaging, how many bleeding, painful bruises did she already have hidden beneath her own cloak?

How beaten down were her hopes, after twelve years of sickness and failed efforts by all the doctors? How much had she been ostracized because of her constant "unclean" state? None of this is mentioned in the Gospel, but we should meditate on the suffering she had endured, the twelve years' time she had lived with her illness and the energy she had spent in searching for a healing. This was a real person. So much had gone on before she reached the climactic moment in the crowd depicted in this Gospel story. Healing takes effort, if only the effort of enduring.

Today, as you awaken with a throbbing pain already in your head, do you wonder, *How long? Why can I not wake up one day feeling "normal" like everyone else, like I used to feel, like I "should" feel?* It may be only ten in the morning, and you have already taken fifteen pills, your stomach is a churning black hole of acid, and the waves of nausea ride up over you as you try to get the vacuum cleaner out of the closet. Your body feels so heavy and weak by midafternoon that you can barely lift your head from the couch. Do others think you're lazy? Only you know the effort it takes to stay in a conversation with your children, your neighbor, or your spouse. Full of guilt once again, you are unable to get to the grocery store or fix dinner. Some cans and packages are left on the kitchen counter, and you are dead away, isolated in bed, again. Is there a miracle in sight? Would it take effort to go in search of one?

In the Gospel story, this woman gathers her strength and puts her hopes into another search. Though Jesus was brought to the homes of many sick people, this woman represents all those who came to him through their pain. She will reach out with her own effort and her own hand to grasp at what she perceives may be the miracle. The Gospels record how she "came up behind him and touched the tassel on his cloak. Immediately her bleeding stopped." She had made it! She had taken steps to come to her healing.

Who knows what she really had expected or how high she had raised her hopes. Who knows what she had felt about this man, Jesus. Was she running to someone she thought of as an alternative-care practitioner or faith healer, in desperation after all the doctors had told her, "You have to learn to live with it"? Or was this more of a spiritual reaching out to a holy man, to simply be near some goodness she had sensed, that she might gain solace in her long suffering? Was this a needy, broken soul, making its best effort to come into contact with the gentle power of pure love and mercy it recognized walking in the crowd?

"'If only I can touch his cloak," she thought, "I shall be cured" (Matthew 9:21). Even if she didn't shout it aloud, she took the risk of being let down again, if only within herself. The point is, she came to the moment open to something new, though her past efforts had left her with disappointment. She invested herself in the process of making something happen, of initiating a change. She took a risk. She invested energy.

She was probably fearful, and she seemed humble. She didn't require a ritual, beyond that of her own reaching out. Maybe she didn't want to bother this man, Jesus, by directly confronting him. Obviously she could have—she had made the effort of working herself all the way through the crowd to touch his cloak. Surely she had the opportunity to look him in the eyes, ask him openly to cure her. But she didn't.

She may have doubted a little, seeming surprised at her cure: "The woman, realizing what had happened to her, approached in fear and trembling" (Mark 5:33). She may have been self-conscious before him and before the others in the crowd who might see her and recognize her. She may have felt foolish for even trying again to find a cure for what had always been deemed incurable. She may have been embarrassed about her very condition, hinted at by the fact that she eventually "fell down before Jesus and told him the whole truth" (Mark 5:33). Certainly even in today's society, it would not be easy for a woman to step out in front of a crowd of strangers to explain a health problem such as this woman had. Perhaps she felt unworthy, so much so that she had to sneak a touch of the power without being noticed, stealing goodness to which she did not feel entitled, yet for which she still hoped.

So often, we are afraid to hope, even secretly, for fear of being let down and disappointed once again. Truly there is energy expended in anticipating, hoping, wanting, and waiting. Energy is also drained by the opposite: dread. True existential fear can lead to our own Gethsemane moments, with a clammy paling of skin and almost sickening light-headedness at the possibility of bad news, loss, illness, death. We don't often know what it is that we truly want, expect, deserve, believe, or fear. All this affects our subsequent responses to events as they then happen.

What was Christ's response to the situation? Here, so far, we have been examining the person who sought healing. What of the healer? When the hemorrhaging woman appears, Jesus was actually on his way to another crisis of illness, a story to be dealt with later.

The initial interpretation of this miracle cure is that Jesus does not have to expend any energy other than what it took to walk through the crowd. Certainly many people touched him that day in the jostle of the crowd: "His disciples said to him, 'You see how the crowd is pressing upon you, and yet you ask, "Who touched me?"'" (Mark 5:31).

There are many other examples in the Gospels where crowds of people came up to touch Jesus. Mark 6:53–56 presents a short description of what sounds like countless cures taking place as people came to him with all their ailments and their sick friends and family. Specifically, they "begged him that they might touch only the tassel on his cloak." All who touched him got well. This same story is conveyed in Matthew 14:35–36, where again "People brought to him all those who were sick and begged him that they might touch only the tassel on his cloak, and as many as touched it were healed."

So, what of our tiptoeing hemorrhaging woman? Why did she garner such a reaction from Christ? Why was her particular touching of just the tassel of his cloak so different from that of all the others?

In Mark, the image of her cure is almost electric—reminiscent of the moment in the movie *Ben-Hur* when the music, light, and emotion swell as the main character's mother and sister are cleansed of their leprosy while Christ is crucified. For the woman in Mark's

Gospel, "immediately her flow of blood dried up. She felt in her body that she was healed of her affliction" (5:29). What an astounding image! She herself was overcome with fear and trembling as she realized what had happened.

True Healing Involves Relationship

But the key line of the story concerns Christ, who was "aware at once that power had gone out from him" (Mark 5:30). Healing is not without cost! It is not without energy, effort, and giving. More important, it is not without relationship. Perhaps it is not without spiritual love on some level. Healing is not a passive event. Part of Jesus had been accessed. The woman's desire to be healed was apparently deep enough to reach Jesus' inherent desire to love and heal; thus she obtained for herself a cure. He says to her later, "Daughter, your faith has saved you" (Mark 5:34).

In this interaction, where is the effort on the part of Christ? It is in the fact that Jesus' entire life was a work of love, an act of his will toward mercy and compassion. His very nature was disposed toward the giving of himself to others. The actions of others touching the tassel of his cloak did not preclude action on Christ's part. The groundwork had been laid by the life Jesus had lived up to that very moment. The Creator has imbued the universe with himself, and each of us with the Holy Spirit, so that from all eternity God's healing love and power are available to us. As a person named Jesus Christ, he had nurtured himself in the love of God throughout his life so that he might be the physical channel for divine love toward humanity. He had predisposed himself to give to the extent that someone, such as this woman, could access his goodness and power, already prepared for her. God's love is always predisposed toward us, waiting to be accessed.

Up to this point in the Gospel story, however, Jesus had not made a personal connection with the woman. She did not grant him the opportunity to reciprocate. All he knew was that someone had touched upon his power.

Jesus needed and wanted to acknowledge this woman as a loved creature and a respected human being. He did not want her to be frightened and embarrassed or guilty at this moment of triumph and wonder. He did not want her to be alone, unable to express her joy at the release from her years of suffering and shame. Perhaps he wanted her to be received back into the community after her years of isolation.

This was not a procedure of modern medical technology performed by a nameless, faceless technician under the aura of sterile blue lights, miraculous as some of those procedures are. This woman did not go into the operating room, about to fall asleep, never having spoken to the world-renowned specialist who would remove her tumor, give her a new heart valve, or relieve her pain. When Jesus engaged the woman, he was making a connection and healing her whole life.

The woman's fears and humility might have cheated that tremendous moment, and Jesus could not let that happen, even on his way to another person in urgent need. He would not go on without making the effort to form relationship. No other person was more important at that time and place than the one who had touched him with her faith and hope. He stopped everything, right then and there, to find the one lost sheep.

The woman had sought Jesus, and Jesus desired to complete the moment. "Jesus . . . turned around in the crowd and asked, 'Who has touched my clothes?'" (Mark 5:30) His disciples were incredulous at his even asking, seeing how dozens or hundreds of people were touching him. Despite this, "he looked around to see who had done it" (Mark 5:32). His efforts must have been so obvious and forceful that we can picture all in the crowd stepping back suddenly, jarred to a hush at his wheeling about.

The woman then presents herself before Jesus and tells "him the whole truth." This perhaps is the honesty and relationship that

Jesus was seeking. He could now give to this individual love and respect. How often does God want to do this with us, while we merely seek to fix a particular part of life that hurts us?

Christ grants to this kneeling, fearful woman the acknowledgment of her great role in the event that has occurred: "Daughter, your faith has saved you." One can hear the emphasis on the word *your,* as much as on the word *faith.* Both are true.

He teaches her to come out in the open and to be a full person in the world from this point forward. This is the resurrecting part of the healing, which makes it far more significant than merely correcting the problem of anemia. He cures her of the greater malady of shame, fear, and whatever else it is that has led her to be secretive in her quest for relief. He is able to send her out into the rest of her life more whole and emboldened. He tells her, "Go in peace and be free of this illness."

Be free. Who can know all that this meant in a time and culture that controlled women, that judged the value of fertility, that feared mysterious, messy, unsightly, and poorly understood disorders? Healing indeed took effort—twelve years of searching on her part; an eternity and a lifetime on Jesus' part.

She went off to the possibilities of her changed life, and Jesus went off to heal the daughter of Jairus, as we shall see later. Perhaps thereafter he was tired, for "he departed from there and came to his native place, accompanied by his disciples" (Mark 6:1). Power had gone from him, and he had felt it.

Healing takes effort, and in true healing there is relationship as well: between the one with the power to heal and the one in need of healing, as well as between individual and community. Healing does not occur in isolation. It may be private, but it involves relationship with God and with others. Our life is different as a result, and we will interact with others and with God differently because of it. God does not demand—not in the Gospels nor in our day—that people pay up for their cures, or that they do something to earn their relief. We must see, in each of the healing stories, that

God wants us to gain much more than what we consciously seek or are even aware of.

We see, throughout the Gospels, that effort is involved in the very nature of seeking God, of enduring the difficulties in life, and of bringing ourselves into contact with God's healing powers. Simply waiting takes effort. So many stories demonstrate the tremendous perseverance of individuals in their suffering and seeking. But perhaps it is partly their own efforts—their searching and perseverance—that solidify their trust in the cure they eventually receive from God. The mystery for us is that God does not toy with us or string us along for his own pleasure or for our punishment. Somehow, healing occurs within the seeking and the effort.

*Oh God, I am so tired and worn by this struggle in which you allow
    me to remain.*
I will keep asking you to ease my burden, Lord.
I know in small ways each day you probably do,
And I ask forgiveness for not seeing that all the time.
I believe you understand when I get frustrated with you,
And when I get sad, and mad, and want to give up.
*I know it is your strength within me that is what keeps me going in
    the first place.*
I want to do great things, Lord.
I want to achieve so much.
It hurts when I am so limited by all that you have given me to bear.
But then, how can I doubt you?
*Somehow, you bear this with me, Lord, for a purpose I cannot
    know.*
I have felt you enough inside me to push on, for you.
*If I can help another by not giving up, I will feel all this is worth it,
    Lord.*
Please grant me the strength to rise to the gift of each new day.
*Let me not be overwhelmed by my pain, my weakness, my sadness,
    or even my anger.*
I look for your tassel in the crowd, dear Jesus.

You know when I find you I will not hesitate to reach out and
touch it.
For I so want to hear those precious words of yours,
"It is your faith that has cured you.
Go in peace and be free of this illness."
Amen

Questions for Your Health

- In health care today, the process of healing can be exhausting and time consuming. When you are aggravated with all the delays in waiting rooms or emergency departments, imagine yourself in the shoes of the hemorrhaging woman, persevering in her long pursuit of Christ.

- Many treatment regimens involve exercises at home, diet restrictions, or lifestyle changes. Do you fully participate in your own care and healing, or do you sometimes neglect your responsibilities? A wise doctor told me what he told his patients: "Look, I did my part; God's doing his part. What are you doing?"

- Ask yourself if you are holding back—in your prayers or in your efforts. Are you willing to risk stepping forward and asking for help? Do not be passive in your relationships with your caregivers. The more you give yourself to them, the more human nature will be called forth in them to work their best for you.

6

"PICK UP YOUR MAT AND WALK."

The Sick Role and What You Do with It

My days pass away like smoke . . . My heart is stricken. . . . Because of my loud groaning my bones cling to my skin. . . . I lie awake. . . . My days are like an evening shadow; I wither away like grass.

Psalm 102 (NRSV)

When I first arrived, the decrepit medical office down at the steel mill was less a care center than a "cauldron of conflict." We were providing occupational medicine, or work-injury care services, for one of America's most well-known industrial giants, and I was to take over for the semiretired doctor who'd been sitting behind a desk there for years. It took one day to figure out the difference between blue-collar work and white-collar work.

The décor was almost what we would picture as early Soviet: gray factory steel and concrete everywhere. The walls were worn cinderblock, the floors either smudged cement or filthy linoleum. The drinking fountains, like the air itself in the building and around it, were covered in a greasy film of settled paint mist, solvents, and grime. A maze of cells made up the medical "clinic." I half expected to follow them back to some room full of torture devices or an ancient leather-strapped electric chair. Remnants of medical equipment did in fact lie about or were crammed into back rooms defaulted to storage—so outdated that we wouldn't think of using them to treat a patient now.

During the first few weeks, I found the medical department to be primarily a place where battles were fought over work releases and job restrictions. Frustrated, screaming plant supervisors called all day long from out in the churning and pounding of the mill, complaining about some lazy, lying lout of theirs who was coming up to try to get himself off work. "And don't you dare fall for it! I need him back down here right away to plug a spot in this shift. I already got two other no-good bums who didn't show up at all." *Click.* Then in front of me would parade a cast of male and female workers who had some pretty impressive ways of presenting their medical cases, most legitimate to a degree, many quite embellished. In the minds of these soldiers of the front lines, their supervisors were generally uncaring, unfair, and uninterested in their pain. The workers in the factory believed no one in management had any concern whatsoever whether they were medically fit to handle the incessant labor demanded of them in the name of increased productivity and higher corporate profits—demands sent from somewhere far away.

Welcome to heavy industry, and big labor, in America. Not quite the perfect environment for spawning intimate and trusting doctor–patient relationships. Into this space came a man and his mat.

Hank, Who Learned to Live Again

The first time Hank walked in, his theatrical persona set him apart from most of the others who waited, wearily slumped in the plastic chairs lined along the dingy narrow hallway. Hank came off as a mix between a biker and an out-of-shape weight lifter. His big belly protruded out from under a tattered purple T-shirt. In fact, he was dressed all in purple, all the time, as I would discover. Beat-up black shoes and too-short worn-out black socks left a little flesh gap beneath what must have been his one pair of torn purple pants. His purple beret was the finishing, European touch.

When the plant nurse, who had been in this pit for more years than she could remember, handed me Hank's chart, she gave it over with an exasperated roll of her eyes. "Here's another winner performing his shtick to earn his time-off job restriction slip, once again." Apparently Hank had been doing this for years, succeeding in getting the prior plant doctor to sign off each time. Sometimes the doctor might have been too lazy to really examine him. Other times he was probably frustrated at a lack of any hint of improvement in Hank's claimed condition, not being able to figure out a way to create a restriction for him, and not being fed up enough to just send him back to work with no mercy and no discussion.

So in he came to me that first time, as had many others, dramatically dragging one leg, limping precariously on the other. It is humorously amazing just how much energy manipulative patients will exert to maintain their injured images. It would be so much less work to slowly walk in and just say that your leg hurts. But that doesn't show the pain enough.

It seemed part of the game in this setting that the patient first had to play out some moves with the doctor in order to win the desired signature on the off-work slip. Some went through the motions cavalierly, remaining laid-back, letting the momentum and inertia of a long list of prior "Fine, you're still off" signatures do the work for them, as had Hank for quite some time now. Others took a more frontal attack, were much more aggressive and intimidating, counting on a fight the moment they stepped in the door. Knowing that this was an encounter with a new doctor, Hank played the role artfully as he told me his tale of woe.

He went round in verbal circles, detailing all his problems from so long ago. He wished he could get better; he wished someone could find a way to help him. Not that he hadn't tried to search for answers. He had seen many doctors, but alas, no one had been able to diagnose him and get rid of his mysterious pain.

Because it had gone on for so long now, his once incredibly active lifestyle was a thing of the past, he assured me. Though I might not believe it, he had been in bodybuilder shape before all of this. Now he calmly lamented his weight gain and poor conditioning. And he confessed that he smoked, too. But when he tried to stop, he would just gain more weight.

Hank appeared to enjoy the intellectual exchange and the telling of his story to this new doctor. I must admit, something about him drew me in. He caught my interest more than most, with their tired stories and attitudes, and mentally I put an asterisk by his name and sent him off without much challenge or threat to change his work status. I did schedule him to come back within a couple of weeks, however, rather than the usual six to twelve months he had expected. He was a little puzzled by that. For the moment, though, he had obtained what he came in for: more time off, tacked onto his running total of three years.

When he came back two weeks later, I spent time delving more into his view of the ailments that disabled him, why he thought it was so hard for the long list of doctors to figure him out. I let him leave again with another time-off slip. But something in Hank's eyes told me he was still reachable. Behind the mask of this injured worker was a glint of honesty. There seemed to be a part of Hank that peeked out cautiously from a distant cave of holed-up self-respect.

Had he wondered how long it would take for someone to find him there? A child hiding in a closet doesn't really want to remain hidden, doesn't want the seeker to quit the game and leave. Would someone take the time, have the nerve, show the interest and compassion to come in after Hank and pull him out of his hiding place? He was willing to be discovered, but it would be too awkward to simply come out on his own. Too much loss of face at this point. And he couldn't merely show up at work better one day, after three years of being too crippled to do anything at all. Someone would have to bring him to that point. Someone would need to cure him first.

So we started to meet regularly and explore ways he could increase, even slightly, his activity level, just to see how much he could tolerate, how we could help him lose weight—but certainly nothing that would entail going back to work. I prescribed a little pain medicine, in case he might occasionally overstrain himself. We talked about the temporary use of an antidepressant at night, just to help him sleep. He wasn't truly depressed, of course, only tired and of low energy during the day, for about a year now. If he slept better at night, his exercise tolerance during the day might improve. He said he really didn't need either type of medicine, but that it might not be a bad idea if it would help him with his exercise.

Hank gradually became more upbeat at his appointments, and not because of the medicines. I think he was starting to live his life better. He said that he was getting around more, doing more things at home, and that his leg wasn't hurting as much. The same nurse was handing me his chart each time but was now raising her eyebrows in wonder.

From the beginning, Hank's eyes had caught me and kept me hanging in there with him. From the earliest versions of his long sob story (which I hate to call it now, but that's what it was), I remained with him, feeling that he and I had the possibility of some tacit understanding. My mind said to his in a respectful yet challenging message: "You've got to be kidding me, Hank. Do you really think I'm going to fall for that line? I won't challenge you now, but know that I know that you're hiding. And more important, you know that you are holding out, way back there somewhere. And by the way, I like you. You seem like a good guy. I think there is so much more to you than what you are revealing. I believe you can walk, that you are not so crippled as you seem."

Well, in the end, Hank pulled himself out of his sick role. He lost all the weight he wanted to. He returned to a program of strength training. He worked with one of our physical therapists to "officially" heal his injured leg ("Finally, someone who knew what he was doing!"). Lo and behold, he suggested he get himself back to work. There was no real explanation for why he hadn't been able to do so before. None was asked for. I gave no real medical explanation for his leg getting better.

His decision to recover was a tremendous risk in many ways, as it is for all patients agreeing to let go of medicines, job restrictions, and court cases after personal injuries. Hank now had to work to get paid. There were no more slips to get him off. He had shown that he was now healthy. And to the end, our eyes stayed connected; he thanked me with his, even as we spoke of mundane things like forms to be filled out. I thanked him with mine, for confirming my faith in him. Neither of us had given up on, nor given in to, the other. He had tested me early on to see if I would be just another person to foster his sick role rather than help him change his life.

He had gotten himself into a bind that he couldn't figure a way out of on his own. He needed someone to help him be healthy again, or the rest of his life would be an act. That's not to say he hadn't had a true medical problem to begin with. But he had become mired in a pattern of passively waiting for someone to push him out. And no one had, so there he remained: a self-limited person in a very boring life. An easy life perhaps, by the standards of those who have to get up and work every day, but nonetheless fruitless and wasted. And he had known it in his soul.

The Man beside the Healing Waters

Now there is in Jerusalem at the Sheep [Gate] a pool called in Hebrew Bethesda, with five porticoes. In these lay a large number of ill, blind, lame, and crippled. One man was there who had been ill for thirty-eight years. When Jesus saw him lying there and knew that he had been ill for a long time, he said to him, "Do you want to be well?" The sick man answered him, "Sir, I have no one to put me into the pool when the water is stirred up; while I am on my way, someone else gets down there before me." Jesus said to him, "Rise, take up your mat, and walk." Immediately the man became well, took up his mat, and walked. (John 5:2–9)

What of this poor fellow who has been waiting for thirty-eight years at the side of a pool that is thought to have healing power? He is there waiting with many others, but Jesus singles him out, or at least the Gospel writers do. We see great fortune bestowed on some and great misfortune on others. Does God pick and choose individuals for suffering or for glory? In point of fact, God singles out each and every one of us, throughout our lives. It is we who too often do not recognize his presence in the stream of events. Even in this story, a few lines later, the man is asked who cured him: "The man who was healed did not know who it was" (John 5:13).

It is interesting how this man answers Jesus' direct question of "Do you want to be well?" He gives an excuse, however legitimate, but an excuse just the same, for why he can't get into the water. If we take an endearing view of this seemingly helpless man, bypassed for years in his hopes of getting into the waters, he is merely lamenting to a stranger that he cannot achieve what he thinks it will take for him to be cured. He has no one to assist him. He valiantly tries on his own but is obviously slow in his efforts, and someone else always gets in ahead of him. The water perhaps moves for only a short time, or maybe there is only a small space where it flows and can be reached. Nevertheless, we can commend him for his diligence. He has not given up after thirty-eight years. He is focused, determined, and steadfast. One day his perseverance may be rewarded. Today is that day, but not in the way he has expected.

Jesus, knowing the situation, offers out of his love, mercy, and limitless compassion to grant this man a new future. He gives him no further hurdles to overcome, no more hoops through which to jump. He sees how hard this man has been striving by himself for years to change his life. The man seems fixated on the pool as his only hope for change; Jesus instead intervenes and grants healing instantly. We can look at this miracle story and see only the instant cure, and wonder why this never seems to happen to us. Or we can see that there is nothing "instant" about an effort of thirty-eight years on the part of this man. Healing takes effort, we see again, if only in the enduring.

When patients despair in how long they've dealt with their maladies or in how they may have to "just live with" their pains into the indefinite future, I remind them that discoveries are occurring all the time, and we never know when a miracle might happen. Just think about this man and put yourself in his position thirty-eight years before we find him in the Gospel story. He perhaps is working and sustains an injury. He could have sustained a spinal cord injury years before and become paraplegic. There are infections of the nervous system such as polio or transverse myelitis, or conditions such as multiple sclerosis and muscular dystrophies that could have made him lame. He might have had some debilitating disorder completely different from paralysis, such as a heart or lung condition that left him with little energy and completely exhausted after the least amount of effort. In any of those scenarios, he could have been left with a miserable life, barely eking out enough to survive, humiliated daily by having to grovel for anything he could get.

Let's say that way back then he asked his doctors how long he'd have to wait to get better. Maybe they said, "We're not sure." Pain is difficult to predict in back injuries. Spinal cord trauma and disease are hard to cure. But let's suppose that they told him to be patient: "Don't worry. In thirty-eight years, a man will come by with a new technique for curing paralysis. You will walk again then." Do you think the man would have been grateful and happy, or terrified and depressed? He would have to wait thirty-eight more years in a paralyzed state, but then he was guaranteed his miracle would occur. Looking at this Gospel miracle from that perspective, perhaps we can see our own waiting for healing in a different light. Not such an instant miracle, was it? The people in these Gospel stories had it no easier than we do.

Lost in a Story of Sickness

Now look at this whole scenario in another light. What if the circumstances surrounding this gentleman's fate were quite different from those laid out above, of a helpless, nobly struggling invalid? Thirty-eight years this man has been there, waiting, as he says, for his chance. But he might have been inattentive to those around him and thus did not care enough about others to connect with them. Maybe people consequently did not like him, did not go out of their way to help him. One can be sick and not very well liked, and come to find, as did this man, that there is never anyone to plunge one into the healing waters, whatever those healing waters may be.

What if we dare to consider for a moment that this man wasn't totally paralyzed at all, at least physically? Like our man Hank at the steel mill, he may have had something happen to him once, thirty-eight years ago. What if he then had become caught up in the illness of it all, trapped in his sick role? And so now he has become this "paralytic" fixture at the poolside. Somehow he has worked out a system of getting himself every day to the pool and then back again to wherever he lives. How, for thirty-eight years (or whatever it was), would he have been able to "get a ride," so to speak, each morning to the pool, be "dropped off," and then picked up again each evening? Yet amazingly, over the same thirty-eight years, he has not been ingenious enough to get someone to take a day or two off work to help him plunge into the pool!

He must have devised some kind of survival network to eat and be clothed. Either he had a supportive family or he was able to beg for money and supplies, obtaining enough each day to get what he needed. He would have been quite well-known around the pool, given how many years he'd lain beside it. It seems odd that no one would notice that this one particular unfortunate man never had anyone available to get him to the waters for at least a try! Maybe he had in fact had offers over the years. Maybe it was he who resisted, graciously of course. This day just wasn't a good day to be moved: "My whole body hurts me too much right now to even be lifted. Oh, that person over there looks to be in much more pain or much worse off; why don't you go help him? Thank you anyway. I've been here so long, I can wait a little longer. I can sacrifice. I can handle it. I'll just do what I've always done. Come back another day, though, and I'll be happy to get well again." If you believe this man to be a real historical person, you have to wonder what he was doing all those thirty-eight years.

Many people may chat with him to be polite, as we often do with street beggars in our own cities. Some leave a coin or two. The very same people, seeing him day after day, might then try to avoid him and his nagging calls for attention, or to avoid having to decide whether to give him more money or more time. The walls built by this man have created walls in others. Thus no one is truly, consistently invested in him. And it is in fact then true that he has no one to help him into the pool.

Then Jesus comes up, knowing this man in some way. Maybe he's heard and seen this man go through his days at the poolside, asking for handouts, resisting offers of help. Perhaps he's exchanged words with the man several times before, as one of the crowd passing by. Perhaps Jesus has given him that look before but bided his time to see what the man would do. In that look, he also might have said, "I like you. I'll be back. We'll talk some more."

On this particular day, in the midst of all the goings-on—the crush of the crowds trying to get into the water, the noise of the splashing, the cries of the beggars, the selling of all sorts of things— picture Christ meeting this man's eyes, penetrating into the soul that is hidden deep within the invalid persona. When Jesus says outright, "Do you really want to be cured?" the man deflects the question, giving not a response but an excuse. Jesus looks piercingly into this man's eyes and listens with compassion, and we can imagine him communicating, through that fastened gaze, "I don't buy it."

What if Christ decided to present the opportunity for a miracle in this man's life, a transformation of his whole way of being? In the secrecy of that tunnel of vision between the two of them, in a silence that blocked out the distraction of human activity around them, did the man recognize the situation: of creature before creator, self-deceit before truth, fear before love?

What if at this moment, after thirty-eight years, the knower-of-all-hearts called forth from the depths of this man a transformation? What if this man, in the sacred space shared between the two of them, perceived Christ's call boring into him, through all his defenses and masks and fears? Go ahead. Do it, my friend! You can! I am giving you the power to give up this half-life, to enter the one God has created for you all along. I am here for you. I will speak the miracle aloud. But the miracle, you and I know, is within you. Stand up, pick up your mat, and walk.

On the one hand, this man is offered freedom and possibility. On the other, that same freedom and possibility represent drastic change and an unknown way ahead. If he stands up now and starts to walk, he cannot go back. What if he isn't able to find a job to support himself? This man, for all we know, has not worked for thirty-eight years! These are the same fears expressed by those in the present-day doctor's office: off work, on disability for months and even years, they are finally told they can go back, or have to go back, to earning a living. This can also be the case for newly divorced or widowed women, who are suddenly left to fend for themselves and perhaps for their children or aging parents, having been out of the workforce for years. What could Jesus have been thinking, forcing this helpless man into the position of having to make such a sudden, all-or-nothing choice?

Remember Christ's words to us elsewhere in the Gospels, when people say to him, "I'll follow you wherever you go but let

me bury my father first," or "I'll be your follower, Lord, but first let
me take leave of my people at home." Jesus responds with the somewhat chilling comment, "No one who sets a hand to the plow and
looks to what was left behind is fit for the kingdom of God" (Luke
9:62). What does he mean when he says this? Is he being dismissive
of humanity's weaknesses? Or is he trying to teach us something
about ourselves?

God's message seems to be that we must let go of the bag-
gage. We are dragged down by our past, our fears, and our self-
protectiveness. We are paralyzed by our overriding attachments to
that which we know, in the face of the future that we do not know.
As we look at the miracle in this Gospel story and wonder how
to apply its message to our lives, we should appreciate the change
asked of this man. He may not even know who he is as a healthy
individual anymore. What is his true identity? He knows only how
to be sick and how to survive being sick.

Yet Christ looks inside, beyond this man's condition, and sees
him full of God's potential yet wallowing in defeat and passivity.
Jesus calls him forth to the risk and to the greatness of something
new. There are no specific instructions. The first step is just that,
the first step.

Ironically, in the Gospel story, the second command of Jesus
to the man, to pick up his mat, gets the man into trouble with
some of the Jews. "It is the sabbath, and it is not lawful for you
to carry your mat" (John 5:10). Isn't it a bit humorous, and sad,
that a man who has not been able to work for thirty-eight years is
immediately castigated by the authorities of the law for "working"
on the Sabbath, the day of his cure, by carrying the mat on which
he has lain invalid for so long? This is another lesson for us as we
look at these miracle stories. Life goes on. People are people. You
will face the same challenges and pettiness in your healing as in
your illness and pain.

As is often the case in the Gospels, Jesus comes back after a
miracle and finds the person whose life has been changed. These

brief reencounters remind us that God does not forget us, nor are we to forget what God has done for us. "Look, you are well; do not sin any more, so that nothing worse may happen to you" (John 5:14).

Jesus is not threatening this man with personal retribution. Nor is he making a direct connection between the man's prior condition and whatever sins he may have had in his life. Jesus wants him to know that a deeper change has taken place beyond the fact that he can physically walk again. Jesus is encouraging the man not to succumb to his fears, not to retreat to some safe but dysfunctional place, thereby losing the gift he has been given. Jesus does not want him to be paralyzed again, this time through his own doubts. He has been granted a healthy wholeness, and Christ desires for him to see beyond the superficial physical aspects of this blessing.

Willing to Get Back into the Game

How many ways do we bind ourselves to our mats? Sickness and pain can intimidate us from taking a risk. We feel too wary of hurting even worse than we already are, or than we have in the past. We may even have recovered significantly from illness or injury, yet we are in no rush to go jumping back into the dangerous and callous game of life. It will demand too much of us and not take into consideration what we have just gone through. We won't get special treatment or sheltering. Life can't be pulled over to the sidelines and told not to hit us too hard, to lay off for a while, seeing that we're still out of shape and a little gun-shy from our recent traumatic experiences.

Sometimes the long suffering of pain or sickness has worn us down. We soften too much, such that *everything* in life hurts, *everything* is too much effort. Even the most mundane and physically non-taxing activities threaten us with discomfort. I am referring to the places we allow ourselves to sink when we have set the bar of life too low, as with our man Hank in the mill or our invalid on his mat. We give up. We stop fighting. We drift down to an imprisoning dysfunctional level. We grant ourselves too many excuses for so many moments of underachieving.

When we are chronically limited by headaches, back pain, obesity, smoking or drug or alcohol habits, anger or bitterness or negativity, it becomes hard to escape the gravity of our own burdens. How is it that we could possibly just get better one day? How could we risk standing up out of the blue, picking up our mats, and walking, as if we were fine? First, we are obviously not fine; second, it would simply be too hard to do, we convince ourselves. The trap can become complex and the inertia profound. Our way of life has revolved around doctors, medicines, surgeries, emergency rooms, and dark, isolated bedrooms. The time off work has been too long to picture going back "in there"—to the office, the plant, the family, the relationship, and all the other demands of life. What we've gone through has been too much, has taken too long, and the way back is too daunting.

While beaten low by our pain, grief, sickness, or dying, are we willing to risk continuing the search for the person who may find us in the crowd, buried yet still alive within ourselves? This is not a half-hearted search either. This is not a muffled call for someone to *kind of* rescue us. This is not looking for codependents or enablers of self-limiting strategies. Rather, it is a search by the courageous for others who would be courageous. It is a quest for genuine insight and true opportunity to be assisted onto our own two feet, literally or figuratively.

We may still have our pain. We may still have a dysfunctional family, or an ornery supervisor, or the bad taste of a lawsuit in our mouths. Jesus says, "Do not turn back once you have placed your hand on the plow with me. Do you wish to follow me, or are you stuck in your old ways? Can you not move beyond what you have lost—even if your loss was an incredible tragedy? Can you not move beyond what you think you deserve or beyond your anger at what has been taken from you?" Christ calls us to walk with him to a new next moment, beyond our present pain and suffering. Do we trust him? Even after thirty-eight years of trying, waiting, surviving? Are we through wasting our lifetimes in bitterness or self-pity or fear-filled excuses?

As was noted at the outset, the more traditional way to look at this healing story is moving and beautiful. For this man and for the valiant people he represents, this story is one of never-say-die hope. Despite all their suffering, they come out into the world each day. They still seek a cure. But it is not available, not possible, not discovered yet. They have not found what or whom they need, and the world of healing has not found them. Someday, somehow, God will find them. Someone will act on their behalf or take the time to solve the puzzle of their problems, or take the chance to finally get to know them. A new surgical technique may be developed. A new medicine may become available. A new love may be possible. And a new life may begin.

The faithful perseverance by the healing waters will not have been in vain. The day when a stranger walks up to them with the miraculous power to say to them, "My friend, your patience has been rewarded. Pick up your mat and walk," will be like heaven. In fullness of faith, for many, that day is the day they reach heaven. Their thirty-eight years may end with God's embrace at heaven's gate: that is no less the miracle, is it?

In the other view of this story, where the man was trapped as a prisoner in his sick role, God does not condemn or castigate, but uplifts and rescues just the same. In both images of the miracle, suffering has been long, and courage to step into the healing is needed. Meanwhile, in the midst of our own "thirty-eight years" of suffering, we are challenged to risk living more in spite of our pain, fatigue, sadness, or waiting for justice. The miracle begins in the courage of connecting with God's eyes that find us, perhaps through another, accepting God's love and receiving that power. At that moment, we start by answering God's call to stand up, pick up whatever mat we've been dependent on, and carry it out of this moment and into a new life.

Pick Up Your Mat and Walk

If you are a beggar on the street,
pick up your mat and walk.
If you are wealthy but not happy,
pick up your mat and walk.
If you have suffered chronic pain and are weary,
pick up your mat and walk.
If you are unhappy in your relationships, or alone,
pick up your mat and walk.
If you have just been told you have cancer and are reeling in your
     shock, don't give up,
pick up your mat and walk.

Pick it up while gazing into the eyes of Christ, midst the busyness
     around you.
Pick it up with his words booming into your heart—come on, dear
     child, you can do it! I know you can. I give you the strength.
Pick it up, even if you still hurt, if you feel tired with that first step.
Pick it up, even when the world calls you a fool or tells you to stop
     hoping for what will never happen.
Pick up your mat and walk, even if physically your condition won't
     let you do it literally—pick it up in your heart, in your attitude, in
     your faith.
Pick it up and walk, dear one, and do not fear the falling, do not fear
     the future, do not fear the risk, do not look back.

You have waited and borne your suffering long enough.
God sees you.
Jesus has found you.
He calls you from your sadness and despair.
He rewards you for your endurance, your patience, your sacrifice,
     your faith.

Stand up.
A new life awaits you.
God wills that it be so.
Pick up your mat and walk!

Questions for Your Health

- The paralytic in the Gospel story was fixated on the pool of water as his only hope of being cured. Then a man came up to him and told him to stand up. Is there something in your life upon which perhaps you have fixed all your hopes? Are you open to the possibility that there is help in places you have not considered, places that others have been suggesting?

- Imagine again that this man was told by his doctor long ago that in thirty-eight years he would be healed. Think of your own situation. Can you take advantage of what medicine and science have to offer you at this moment, and live with the hope that greater things are always possible?

- In what ways have you perhaps paralyzed yourself beyond the true limits of your disease? Is there anything "good" about remaining so paralyzed?

- What is the most frightening thing about getting better and trying to resume a more normal life? Are there ways your doctor, your family, or your employer can help allay your concerns about "getting back into the game"?

7

"THE CHILD IS NOT DEAD BUT ONLY ASLEEP."

The Trust That Takes You Farther Than Fear

Do not let the flood sweep over me, or the deep swallow me up, or the Pit close its mouth over me.

Psalm 69 (NRSV)

Isn't it amazing that, no matter how much we proclaim our faith or how often we have experienced the very presence of God in our lives, we can still so quickly and completely dissolve into panic and fear when something goes wrong? We receive a call that a medical lab result has come back abnormal and that more tests need to be done. One's wife returns from a visit to her gynecologist to report that a lump was found in her breast. An energetic man, after nearly five years of being cancer-free, is suddenly fatigued. A CAT scan shows the mass has returned; it is treatable, but the memories of the harrowing, painful course of radiation, chemotherapy, and surgical recovery are overwhelming.

What of situational bad news in our lives? We lose a job, or a relationship goes sour. One's life savings account starts to plummet under poor money management in an economic recession. Credit card bills come in the mail with disastrously high amounts due, at the same time the car payments, the rent, and the gas and electric bills have to be paid. The phone company is threatening to turn off service. You won't be paid for another two weeks. A son keeps getting into trouble at school and doesn't talk when he's home in his sullen, distant moods. A daughter, sick of all the rules her mother throws at her, disappears for two weeks. Your back is killing you. Your headache is blinding. Everything is whirling out of control.

A Little Girl Almost Lost

> Part of the pain of life for parents lies in the fact that they cannot protect their children from life. No mother can warn them sufficiently or hope even to be understood if she tries. Nor can she suffer for them. Parents can only do their best and set their children free to encounter existence on their own. (Eugene C. Kennedy, *The Pain of Being Human*)

Jeanette was only twelve years old when disaster came to her and her parents. She lay there unconscious on the ball field, bleeding— possibly dead or paralyzed. The dreaded unthinkable disaster had happened. Her parents stared at their child lying on the ground, not moving. The bat had hit her in the head so hard that the crowd gasped aloud as one at the ugly stomach-turning sound. She dropped like a porcelain vase falling off a table.

The coach and trainers were all huddled over her now. Mom and dad climbed past everyone, pushing through the hushed crowd that looked at them and then back at the place where the little girl lay. Tears clouded their eyes even as they fought the scenes racing through their minds of a hospital intensive care unit, surgery, a funeral—oh, God, no, not that! Save her, save her, please! Oh, don't let her be hurt badly, dear Lord; she's too young, she's too little, she's our precious daughter!

That was more than a year ago. Amazingly, little Jeanette survived. It was scary for a while, that first week in the hospital, with two surgeries to fix the skull fracture and plastic surgery to repair the gash in her forehead. She was beautiful as ever, with hardly a scar at all.

But Jeanette's parents had never quite gotten over that dreadful moment and the first few days of wondering whether they had lost their daughter. Even in the emergency room, seeing that she was not going to die, they feared that she would be crippled or brain damaged for life. Her rapid recovery was a giddy miracle to them, but they subconsciously remained haunted by the shock of those first few moments when she lay limp in the dirt. They had not dealt with the insecurity that had entered their lives when they witnessed how suddenly life could change, how quickly all dreams and happiness could be lost, destroyed.

In the intimacy of communication between parents and children, Jeanette sensed that she was somehow different now to her parents. She was more fragile. She had to be watched over, protected. Wordlessly it had been conveyed to her through her parents' subtle nervousness that she was still in some kind of danger.

At home, with mom and dad treating her more like a three- or four-year-old, Jeanette started to feel confused about not being such a big girl anymore. After all, when out with her peers, life had gone way beyond the world of toddlers. To be sure, she was still having some headaches and neck pain, but nothing neurologically serious. Nevertheless, her parents couldn't help worrying, and they seemed to be searching for something much more sinister and evil that had to be uncovered and eradicated before it took Jeanette away. It had failed the first time on that awful day, and here it was sneaking back again to steal her before their very eyes. Couldn't anyone else see what was happening? Someone needed to figure this out before it was too late.

Meanwhile, Jeanette was caught up in the intrigue, childishly dizzy with the mysterious power she had discovered, which could turn an adult's world upside down. And that was the problem: the normal parent—child dynamics were spiraling into a seriously dysfunctional state, which did risk truly affecting this little girl's life from a psychological, developmental perspective. Jeanette and her parents had been granted their miracle way back in those first few days after the accident. Now they had to trust in it. But they were afraid.

The Temptation to Panic

There are many examples of situations where people cry out, helpless in their anxiety and panic at all that seems to be going wrong. Patients and their families come in completely at their wits' end, for example, because pain is out of control and the medicines aren't working or are causing so many side effects. Even the treatments available are surrounded by complicating issues. Some could get surgery but are too afraid of the risks; meanwhile, they can't stand in the kitchen long enough to make a meal, so severe is the spinal stenosis. Others are in the midst of tons of stress at work, and now is not a time that they can just take off to rehabilitate, even though their pain is unbearable. There are wives who must remain in abusive relationships because they are dependent on the insurance coverage through their husbands' jobs in order to get the therapy and treatments they need. There are children and teenagers who must create whole worlds of survival in order to make it through the years they must live with an alcoholic parent, and the stress grows into headaches, ulcers, or asthma.

Each of us fears the possibility that one day we will be diagnosed with cancer. Tom came in with a minor problem of a bothersome backache. He thought it was the result of having awkwardly lifted a lawn mower months ago, but it wouldn't go away and had become more and more nagging. It wasn't bad during the day, but at night it always bothered him, to the point that he couldn't find a comfortable position for sleep. He received some physical therapy but wasn't making any real progress with the usual treatment plan. His therapist then sent him to me.

The person I met was a bright, physically fit man, a husband and father with a great personality. He told me his story, and we went through a very detailed neurologic, orthopedic, and spinal exam. My concerns were raised by what he did not report in his history and by what I could not find upon examination. He did not have any of the usual symptoms, patterns, or signs common to disc or joint problems, pinched nerves, or strained muscles. What he did have was the red flag of pure nighttime pain. His exam had some odd components to it. Not to alarm him, I told him that he might have a disc problem but at an unusual level in his spine. The larger concern, unvoiced at that point, was whether he had something more serious that might have been unmasked several months before with the innocuous lifting of a lawn mower.

My suspicion was well-founded, as the MRI that I ordered revealed a large spinal tumor. I knew that Tom was not in the least anticipating such news. There is no easy way to blunt the impact of words like "mass" or "tumor" or "growth" when first having to convey them to a patient. One does not have to use the term *cancer* at all to produce a chilling effect of shock and dread, fear and near panic. I could see this poor young man go white and almost faint as his mind registered what he was hearing. It is difficult to explain much at such moments, even in order to allay unnecessary fears, because the psyche of the patient has alarms going off everywhere. The person can't even hear the doctor's words; he is too busy fighting the sudden, overwhelming nausea. Tom lay down his head and tried to get a grip so he could stay focused.

In the end, he made it through that first meeting. His wife was out of town, and he had to return home to take care of his two young rambunctious boys. He received more tests, went for second opinions, and was able to gather himself courageously for his surgery. He actually had a good prognosis despite the delicate nature of the surgery necessary on his spinal cord. Short of dying from cancer, the other primary dread of most patients is that they will become paralyzed from their illness or from a surgery. Tom had all those things to worry about. But he held on, regained control of the ship, and rode out the storm with amazing composure.

Another patient, Miguel, wasn't so strong on composure. He had bad luck with his back and, unfortunately, had been through five spine surgeries by the time I saw him for the first time. He was in terrible pain and still wanted something done, desperately. He did not have a quiet space in his life or in his mind. He externalized his anxieties and gave over responsibility and control to anyone who would take them from him. In his panic, he would react to any procedure, even the most minor ones, with displays of incapacitating pain. He insisted on immediate relief with strong pain medicines and overnight hospital stays.

This kind of patient is often the one who gets himself into deeper trouble, because in his desperation he allows people to do too many procedures on him. He has only one thought in mind: to find someone who will make all the pain go away. This is a slippery slope of one doctor after another trying to rescue him with more well-intentioned surgery, increasing the risk of complications or longer-than-usual postoperative pain. The patient panics about the possibility of something else now being terribly wrong, and another procedure is done to correct or supplement the first, and on down the slope it goes.

When I saw Miguel, I placed him in the hospital for some aggressive pain-medicine treatment in order to get him settled down. He actually seemed to get worse when he should have been getting at least a little better. I had to take the risk of having a heart-to-heart talk with him about how I believed that it was his reaction to pain that was getting him into more and more trouble.

In a quiet space, late in the evening, we had a talk about how, with our assistance, he had to begin a course of care that would aid him in managing his own fears as well as his very real pain. He needed to accept that he was five surgeries in the hole, and that in all likelihood he had to reevaluate how he was going to live the rest of his life. He was forty-three and wanted everything to be just like it used to be. He was fixated on how "screwed up" he was, how much of "a mess" he was in. It was extremely difficult to get through to him with all the clamor and noise in his own mind. I told him, after ascertaining somewhat his faith life, that he needed to quietly give his fears and disappointments and wild imaginings over to God, and to ask for the courage and the composure to reenter his life day by day.

Already he had been to more doctors than was good for him, and was stuck with the consequences. He could not get mired in regret and lament. I offered him the hope that we had some advanced procedures to manage his type of pain, but I also warned him that we could not get caught in the trap that had landed him in this situation: that of chasing after cures in desperate attempts to rescue him, potentially adding more problems rather than alleviating any. I needed him to work with me, to settle down in his demeanor and responses to his everyday discomforts, so that we could discern what was serious and what wasn't. I realize that it is a lot easier, however, to be at the *side* of the bed, saying those words, than it is to be *in* the bed, trying to heed them.

Where is God in the midst of our panic? Don't we all wonder if he hears our cries? When life seems so utterly crushing and painful and cruel, how is it that God doesn't let us know he is there? And if he is there, why doesn't he just fix the problems, rather than allow us the torture of suffering through them? We don't want lessons; we want relief. We want to be rescued. We bang fruitlessly on the doors of heaven. Does he not hear, or does he not care? Or is he really just not even there?

Searching outside the Box

How far outside the box are we willing to go for our own healings? Too often, we find only what we expect to find, and in the place where we expect to find it. We negate that in which we have been taught not to believe.

How do we recognize the boxes we live in? In the United States, it has taken quite a long time for doctors and patients to be open to options such as acupuncture, magnet therapy, mind–body relaxation and creative techniques, and other nontraditional therapies. MRIs are ordered every day by the thousands—they are *magnetic* resonance imagers. Not too much of a problem using magnets there. Ocean tides can move forty to sixty feet twice a day in some parts of the world. Can we not accept that small changes in barometric pressure—the weather—can move tiny molecules of water in our joints and tissues and make us achy and miserable? Countless drugs act on positively or negatively charged parts of chemicals or cell structures in our bodies. Why the doubt about acupuncture's use of simple conductive metal needles inserted into the "battery" of our bodies, fluid-filled containers of charged molecules and electrolytes? Perhaps we don't feel they are big enough, complex enough, technological enough, or expensive enough to handle the perceived complexity of the disorders we have.

The body and its dysfunctions—pain in particular—can be accessed, evaluated, and treated in many ways, most not mutually exclusive of one another. In this way, the body is like the universe: it can be seen with light telescopes or heard with radio telescopes. The universe really doesn't care, nor is it fundamentally any different as a result of which type of device or which sense organ we use to describe it. The universe is what it is. The question is whether the observers are open to learning in different ways.

We may not always be able to see or understand the help that is available to us. We may resist because something seems too familiar or too foolish. We may refuse to try something because we don't like who is offering us the help or how the help and suggestions are being offered. We may be embarrassed to admit we've changed our minds, or that our own efforts have not gotten us very far or that we are simply weak, and desperate to be relieved of our misery. Whatever the reason, at some point in our search for healing, we will probably have to face the challenge to step out of the boxes in which we live 90 percent of our lives. It will often be a leap of faith.

The air all around us is invisible and silent, until we push a button on a box and see television images on a screen or hear music on a radio or a person's voice on a phone. It just depends on which antenna we stick up into the empty air and activate. The images, music, and voices are always there in the seeming emptiness around us. Thus it is with the possibilities of pain management. Are you willing to admit that there exist answers, options, techniques, and resources about which you are not even aware? The Spirit is all around us, and healing is in the air, if we are but open to access it, in ways we may not expect to. Step out of the box. Put up another antenna. Change the station if you have to until you find a voice you can work with.

The Daughter of Jairus

One of the synagogue officials, named Jairus, came forward. Seeing him he fell at his feet and pleaded earnestly with him, saying, "My daughter is at the point of death. Please, come lay your hands on her that she may get well and live." He went off with him, and a large crowd followed him and pressed upon him. . . .

While he was still speaking, people from the synagogue official's house arrived and said, "Your daughter has died; why trouble the teacher any longer?" Disregarding the message that was reported, Jesus said to the synagogue official, "Do not be afraid; just have faith." He did not allow anyone to accompany him inside except Peter, James, and John, the brother of James. When they arrived at

the house of the synagogue official, he caught sight of a commo-
tion, people weeping and wailing loudly. So he went in and said to
them, "Why this commotion and weeping? The child is not dead but
asleep." And they ridiculed him. Then he put them all out. He took
along the child's father and mother and those who were with him
and entered the room where the child was. He took the child by the
hand and said to her, "Talitha koum," which means, "Little girl,
I say to you, arise!" The girl, a child of twelve, arose immediately
and walked around. [At that] they were utterly astounded. He gave
strict orders that no one should know this and said that she should
be given something to eat. (Mark 5:22–24, 35–43)

What does Jesus come upon when he encounters the situation above? It seems a near riot of hysteria. Though perhaps it was a custom in that culture to wail over a death, even Jesus is taken aback, saying to the crowd, "Why this commotion and weeping?" And what is Jesus' response to this scene? He enters a more intimate space with the girl's parents and his own friends and gently asks her to wake up. He enters a crisis and brings peace. He teaches us to remain calm amidst our confusion and fears.

Do we allow him space in our hearts, our lives, our crises and fears? If we are quiet beyond our own panicking and wailing thoughts, we may be able to notice that Jesus has already arrived. If we have trust, we may be able to accept as helpful something that at first seems a ridiculous solution to our perilous, hopeless situations. The crowd in the story can only see what they expect to see. They have made up their minds and behave accordingly. They give up and say, "Don't bother the teacher." It is not wrong that they react with grief at the first news of the little girl's death. Yet the insinuation by the Gospel writer is that they are guilty of something more disturbing. Jesus is amazed by the level of the reaction. Is there something insincere in the crowd? Is there complete faithlessness in the goodness of God, even though a child has died? Not only that, they are certainly able to compose themselves quickly enough to stop and argue with him.

An Invitation to Wait Quietly

I do see patients who are so deafened by the din in their minds that they don't allow for a quiet awareness of what may be possible. Jesus asks you for the faith to toss your nets out again, despite your long night of catching nothing. He doesn't always instantly "cure" us, rescue us, or save us from the ongoing circumstances. He knows what we need at each moment, if we are willing to trust in the gift, even though it seems too small to make a difference before our towering fears. He does sometimes have to redirect us in our frenetic search for answers or call our attention when we are caught up in our own lamenting.

Like children, we can be so lost in our crises that we doubt the possibility of miracles. Christ is always available. We need only to invite him in, as Jairus did. It helps if we have trust. In the Gospel story, Jairus has to wait for Jesus to make it through the pressing crowd. This is where Jesus encounters the woman with the hemorrhage in the story we explored earlier, when he felt power go out of him. The desperate father had to wait for Jesus to work his way through the world around him. Meanwhile, his little girl was dying. Though we all want to be generous with others and to have God attend to the suffering of all, when it is ourselves or someone we love who is in a crisis, it is hard to wait for God.

Think of a wailing child who seems unreachable, determined to get in a good, eye-scrunching, earsplitting cry. In the end, we hold him, calm him down, soothe his brokenness, and let him feel the presence of love and safety. God is all-wise, aware of human nature. God knows that sometimes we need the tangible touch and the saving ritual. When Jesus was on earth, he could walk through the wailing and take a little girl by the hand. Now he acts through each of us. We are asked to bring peace to one another, and we are also asked to accept peace from others when we need it.

We may be praying and crying for the great cure while not receiving—or even seeing—all the little cures being generously given to us each day. Healing and miracles do not usually come in all-or-nothing cures. One doesn't usually awake on a Tuesday morning, after years of suffering, to find that all pain has completely disappeared. Have I seen this happen? Yes. Does it happen often? No.

Sacred Spaces and Words That Save

There are some patients who come in as one of the four endearing characters in the great classic *The Wizard of Oz,* caught up in the drama of their search for a cure. Each character is convinced that he or she is in need of some vital, profound aspect of life, presently missing, that if found and provided would make life complete at last. Beyond broomsticks, wicked witches, flying monkeys, and the conjured-up figure of a great and powerful, fire-and-brimstone Oz, the four come to a quiet, intimate moment with a man behind a curtain. He has the insight to sense their needs, fears, disappointments, and disillusions. He genuinely sees into each of their lives and gives them gifts that release the fullness of life already within them. They, in turn, are open to receiving the gifts they seek, via the ritual of the tangible symbols bestowed on them by this wise man. In the words of the Scarecrow: "Oh joy! Rapture! I've got a brain!"

The man doesn't merely tell them they are fine, to quit panicking and wailing, and to go on their ways. He meets each of them in the emptiness he or she feels. He touches them in that sacred space. Doctors, nurses, therapists, and family caregivers should learn from this: We can't simply send patients away, telling them they are fine when they are clearly convinced that they're not. At the same time, it doesn't help to chase after esoteric medical diagnoses if they are not truly indicated. A thorough doctor will quietly pursue all possible avenues of cause for illness, while fostering as much health and confidence and calmness in the ill person as is appropriate and possible.

God does work through each of us. Therefore, risk faith in that doctor, nurse, or therapist who comes quietly into your room. Pray to discern God's presence in these helpers. Jairus put his trust in Jesus— and it's doubtful that he possessed the theological insight to believe Jesus to in truth be the incarnate Creator God. Jairus was a human being like each of us, caught in a moment of desperation, seeking help where he thought it could be found. Even while those around him were losing their composure, he held onto a sense of the possible that he must have perceived in the unflustered demeanor of Jesus. When greeted at his home with the news that his daughter had already died, Jairus chose to keep his eyes on Christ. He also kept his eyes on the little girl he loved, and for her sake he was deterred neither by the crowd nor by what might have been his own doubt and fear.

So tightly do we hold onto the demand for answers sometimes that we are unable to grasp the calming words of God, perhaps because they are offered too simply through the people around us. Our problems have defeated so many before—the brilliant doctors, the high-tech procedures, the wonder drugs—that we wail inconsolably at our cruel fate and assume that we are beyond rescue.

When we are ill or in pain, it often takes the touch of someone with power, love, and assurance to get us out of our sickbeds. Even the act of allowing someone to touch us where we have been hurt takes a lot of trust, and usually trust takes time. Trust allows us to listen, to wait, and to be led by our God to a deeper place, where healing can happen.

We may want to be independent or strong. We want to be able to overcome pain, to suppress it, to make it go away. Unfortunately though, just as we don't yet know how to tell our livers to stop making so much cholesterol or our pancreas to make more insulin, we can't make our muscles stop hurting, our heads stop pounding, our backs stop aching, or our nerves stop shooting pains. We can't make our paralyzed legs move, or our stroke undo itself so that we can talk again. We can't stop our depressions and our sorrows, and we can't bring back a lost love or loved one.

In the novel *The Horse Whisperer,* a young girl must be healed of her own physical losses from a terrible injury, as well as of her relationship losses. Her horse was badly injured along with the girl, and in their woundedness the two are estranged from each other. A stranger arrives who seems to have special powers with horses. Through those powers, he is able to influence the healing of the girl beyond her physical scars. As an allegorical vehicle, we can see the injured horse as our own injured body. The girl sitting on the horse is our mind. Sometimes body and mind are disconnected in injury and disease, and we can't seem to find the answers, despite all our well-intentioned searching. We must give over control and let someone work on us, until we can climb back up and be whole again, even if in a different way than we were or than we originally wanted.

I send patients to therapists with that message. Let the miracle happen by such mundane first steps. Allow your body to be touched, the pain to be accessed. Let the hurt be soothed and all the pent-up anger and frustration be vented. Trust that physical and psychological walls can be dismantled from around you if you allow yourself to give over a little control. You are that child in *The Horse Whisperer.* Let yourself stand back at first while the expert calms the skittish, suspicious animal that is your body. Just as the horse must give itself over to the hand of the trainer, so your body must be given over to its healer.

You have within you the faith that will be your salvation. Do not undervalue the gifts given you each day in the form of those around you. Do not look so hard beyond what is right in front of you, and do not get caught up in the fear and the wailing, whether in your own mind or in the world around you. God knows what you need at each moment and has given you the power and resources to sustain you through these trials. God does not say there will be no suffering. But God will never arrive too late to save you. Your faith can be your salvation. Christ says to us in this story of Jairus that he is with us, despite the appearance of hopelessness and loss. When our minds are swirling in the middle of the night with all sorts of fears and scenarios that leave us in near panic, he says, "I am coming. I know where you are. I will not be too late to save you. You are feverish in your concerns over what has gone wrong in your life. You are worried about your finances, growing old, not being married, or not having children. You are frightened of what will become of you. You are fearful of failure and embarrassment. Your debts are piling up. Your addictions are too strong for you. Your pain is devouring you. You beg for the cup to be taken from you as your kidneys fail and no transplant is yet available. I am ever in pursuit of you while you run in fear, lost in your own despair. Come with me to a quiet sacred space."

In that sacred space, the intimate circle that includes ourselves and the healing presence of God, we can find a way even through tragedy. We can learn to quiet our rage and frustration enough to hear Jesus and feel his hand upon us. Christ, through someone or something, takes hold of us and gently says, "Get up."

My God, my God, do you know my pain?
I cry like the psalmist that you have left me here to die.
What is the reason, what is your purpose—
How can it be good, when this is surely so bad?
I want to feel you rescuing me from your cross.
I want to scream for you to save me from this.
But then I feel the guilt and the shame.
I am broken, O Lord.
I cannot help but admit it.
I am fearful this will never end.
Do you care?
Do you hear me?
Are you there?
I want you to be.
I need you to be.
Find me, O God.
I cry, but I will wait for you.

Questions for Your Health

- In the midst of all the stresses surrounding your out-of-control pain, or your struggle with a decision about a difficult treatment plan, whose is the calmest voice in your life? Is it that of your doctor, your spouse, a minister, a friend, your attorney? Give yourself time and space with that person so that you can more clearly move forward through this fearful phase.

- When it is your own soul that is in a panic, fearing that all may be going wrong—in your life or in the life of someone you love—how do you find a place in which to hear God's voice? Have you tried to make a habit of stopping at a church or chapel for a half hour of peace each day? Are you able to go for a walk or listen to calming music on headphones perhaps? If you are Catholic, do you take advantage of meditating through the rosary or the stations of the cross? Can you watch the sunrise each morning and ask God's peace for the coming day? Do you write in a journal to empty your head of its whirling thoughts?

- Breathing well is so simple, yet deep breathing is the foundation of so many therapies, meditation and relaxation techniques, visualization practices, and prayer. If nothing else, in the midst of panic or pain, breathe slowly and fully. Let the spirit of God wash through you. It may not take much of the pain away, but it is at such moments that you most need to acknowledge the spirit of God within you. The Spirit will instruct you on the rest. Breathe. . . .

8

"STRETCH OUT YOUR HAND."

The Innocent Who Suffer in Silence

I am utterly bowed down and prostrate; all day long I go around mourning. . . . I am utterly spent and crushed. . . . My hearts throbs, my strength fails me. . . . For I am ready to fall, and my pain is ever with me.

Psalm 38 (NRSV)

Iris had suffered her headaches for twenty-two years. Her identity had essentially become one with her pain, and every day was infused with at least some level of discomfort. Even on what she might consider a good day, a low throb ebbed and flowed deep in the chambers of her head. On a bad day, the crushing on her skull was merciless and made her stagger. The muscles of her neck and shoulders were embedded with hard, burning rocks, buried so far within her that they had become part of her back's terrain. She knew the familiar hand that reached to the nape of her neck, applying its iron grip, then locking itself under the base of her skull. If only at this moment she could separate her skull from the top of her neck. They were too close together, too compressed and jammed. The hardness of the pain generated there would soon become a diamond drill pushing out through her forehead.

But the pain never vented itself. No wonder ancient cultures used trephines—saw-toothed cylinders—to cut holes in skulls in hopes of relieving the evil humors of crazed sufferers. The inward rushing pain had nowhere to go. An invisible vise around Iris's head squeezed at her temples, keeping the pain trapped. She could hardly see out through the hazy zone of pain that enveloped her. Dazed, staggering, and disoriented, she was disconnected from the details around her. Yet the lights, sounds, and odors were magnified and felt like reverberating hammers. The mere effort of holding up her head or keeping her eyes open to pay attention to a person talking to her taxed her to exhaustion. Thinking and listening were absurdly burdensome expenditures of energy. Regardless of her desire to tough it out, at these moments she could only concede to the power overwhelming her.

What of all those times when she wanted to have guests over, or agreed to go out to a dinner party with her husband, or was supposed to babysit the romping, crying grandchildren? Was it her fault that these incapacitating days would then come on, disabling her beyond any desire to go on with everyday plans? Had she tried to do too much the day before, ignoring her own warning signs? But she was sick of doing nothing, and on a relatively good day she wanted to pretend she was normal. Was that a bad thing? She shouldn't act fragile all the time, should she? Or was this just denial, which in the end exacted its price from her and from those who made plans involving her?

She felt that others blamed her for being too stressed, or angry, or depressed, bottling all this inside a skull too small and inelastic to bear it. Yet she had always tried to be as pleasant as possible, not complaining, suppressing the dull roar of pain that, truth be told, was now present in each day of her life. Others could not see the invisible demons plaguing her, as she looked out from within her isolating cloud. They couldn't know the battles she fought each day to appear as if life were fine, as if mundane tasks were easy, that a ride in the car to the store was not a major decision to weigh.

She *was* stressed, angry, and depressed. Even this was hard for her to admit to herself, so fine was the balancing line between fighting off the pain and acknowledging it, giving in to it when she was forced to concede to its dominance over her. Why did she have to have it? Why couldn't all the headache experts and their clinics and brain scans detect something? "Chronic daily headache with migraine variants" was the diagnosis she was awarded. And all the negative test results: MRI, MRA, CAT, PET—they seemed to proclaim that she was making it all up and that she was somehow weak in dealing with life.

And the medicines they poured into her—that dulled her, sickened her stomach, or made her light-headed when she tried to stand up. She could not tolerate those that came even close to alleviating some of her pain. But these were all that were available as far as she knew; she could only trust what her doctors told her. She was weary of trying new techniques. They often hurt more than they helped. She grew disappointed when they didn't work—not that they didn't help a little sometimes, but against the monster of her pain, they seemed so insubstantial.

She felt like a tiny figure, sitting on a long flat beach at the water's edge, looking to the roaming, undulating ocean of pain stretching its vastness before her. At any moment, this ocean could just reach out and swamp her. It was always there: mighty, deep, endless, impassive, inescapable. It was her pain. How could she defeat it? Who could empty it, drain it away from her? Even if the tide were out a while, giving her a little sense of space between herself and her pain, it would always come back—that's how oceans are; that's what oceans do, even oceans of pain. "My God, my God, why have you forsaken me?" she would cry, and then feel guilty. "Just let me die," she would say, giving in. And then she would feel even more guilty.

How could she complain? Wasn't there suffering everywhere? She was able to walk. She had her vision and her hearing. She still had her mental capacities, her memory, her ability to think, to pray. She lived in a good home, in a rich country. She recognized that she was so much better off than a lot of other people. She didn't have cancer. She wasn't dying, but she felt quite dead. Her cross was invisible. She tried to bear within herself the crown of thorns and the rough weight on her shoulders. *But how long, O Lord, how long?* She almost wanted to say the blasphemous: "But your pain, God, was only for one day, for a matter of hours." *God forgive me, how could I even think . . . I surely deserve even more pain now. How could I dare to even equate mine. . . .*

It is all right to lament. It is all right to sob, break, and surrender. The Bible is full of cries to God out of the depths of sorrow, loss, despair, and fear. The history of earth is awash with the rage at what was allowed to be, the maddening frustration at the rescues and relief never delivered. We are bent not only by the burden of suffering but also by the self-imposed guilt of not bearing it as saintly as we tell ourselves we should, were we better people or our faith stronger.

A Woman Ill for Eighteen Years

> A woman was there who for eighteen years had been crippled by a spirit; she was bent over, completely incapable of standing erect. When Jesus saw her, he called to her and said, "Woman, you are set free of your infirmity." He laid his hands on her, and she at once stood up straight and glorified God. (Luke 13: 11–13)

We don't know what was going on within the mind of the woman bent over for eighteen years. Had she felt she was paying for some sin? Had she been overburdened with spinal arthritis or perhaps with accumulated disappointments? Perhaps she might never have recovered from the loss of a child, a spouse, a love, or a way of life. Whether she had osteoporotic compression fractures, Parkinson's disease, or a psychological depression, it does not matter. Chronic pain will wear down the sufferer.

Pain is such an insidiously crushing "disease" to carry. It is usually believed to be a symptom and sign of some underlying wrong.

We don't often think of pain as a disease, in and of itself, as we do high blood pressure, diabetes, thyroid disorders, muscular dystrophy, or cancer. Pain lives wherever we do. It can bend us low under its burden. Pain can empty us of our very spirit, draining us of our strength. It does not show up on MRI scans or blood tests. Surgeons cannot see it when they open up the body.

Under the barrage of unremitting pain, the nervous system can lose its resilience. Its backup coping mechanisms are dissipated of their norepinephrine and dopamine neurotransmitter fuel. Interneurons within the spinal cord are reprogrammed into distorted hypersensitized pain generators that fire independently of actual continued tissue damage elsewhere in the body. In other words, the initial cause for pain may be gone, but the body continues to register pain anyway. The result may be the pain of Iris's now daily headaches. There are many other types of central pain syndromes, along with the more peripheral neuropathic pain phenomena in diabetics and alcoholics. The will and spirit can be drained to the point that literally or figuratively each becomes "completely incapable of standing erect." We can become so fatigued and despairing that we're unable to notice the saving presence of anyone, much less God.

Christ is often shown in the Gospels to be moved with pity at the sight of someone buried in his or her sorrow, pain, or guilt. These particular people do not call or shout to him for a cure. Instead Jesus is drawn by his own compassion to discern the quiet suffering in the crowd. These suffering people may be lamenting within their hearts and prayers while bearing their sorrows silently. Christ notices even those too broken to interact with the world any longer, and he reaches out to touch and save them. We see analogies to this on our own streets with regard to the homeless and beggars. There are those with lots of energy, endlessly hounding each passerby, hawking for money. There are others, though, so lost and withdrawn from life that they just sit in heaps against buildings or search garbage cans in slow motion, oblivious to any possibility of help around them.

Does Christ become upset with those who beg for mercy and relief from a sincere heart? Absolutely not. But he sees those numbed into submission and silenced by their pain. Ironically, Christ is accused of breaking the Sabbath in performing this miracle. He says to the chief of the synagogue in the story of the woman, "This daughter of Abraham, whom Satan has bound for eighteen years now, ought she not to have been set free on the sabbath day from this bondage?" (Luke 13:16). He is demonstrating and assuring us that God cannot and will not "rest" when there is suffering before him. Thus Jesus "works" on the Sabbath to heal a suffering woman. We don't know what he means by saying this woman had "been in the bondage of Satan." Whatever we name evil and suffering in the world—this bondage of Satan over us—Christ will not leave us helpless.

A Man with a Withered Hand

> *Again he entered the synagogue. There was a man there who had a withered hand. They watched him closely to see if he would cure him on the sabbath so that they might accuse him. He said to the man with the withered hand, "Come up here before us." Then he said to them, "Is it lawful to do good on the sabbath rather than to do evil, to save life rather than to destroy it?" But they remained silent. Looking around at them with anger and grieved at their hardness of heart, he said to the man, "Stretch out your hand." He stretched it out and his hand was restored. (Mark 3:1–5)*

My brother, Michael, has a "shriveled hand," or a "withered hand" as it is also described in the Gospels. It is small and preciously soft. It is vulnerable and weak. It is not fully useless, though, and thus has an individual character of its own. It is valiant in its effort to assist, to do its part for its owner and for its own stronger brother on the other side. Michael was born with that hand the way it is; in fact, his whole right side is weaker than his left, smaller and less muscled. But it is his hand that captures the eye. It is clasped fervently by his stronger hand as he prays with tightly closed eyes. It does its best to make the sign of the cross, dutifully following everyone else's right-handed sign of the cross. It reaches out disarmingly, so to speak, to those around him at Mass during the handshake of peace, as he genuinely gives them his best blessing, face beaming at the chance to connect with another person. With much effort, it holds down the end of a shoelace while his left hand manipulates the other lace. It patiently gets mittened by its stronger other half, but does its darnedest to help the left hand with its own mitten in the windy biting cold of a bus stop. It bears the marks of scrapes and scratches from being fallen on or banged against. It can even almost straighten itself when asked, but only with tremendous effort and with each finger a little crooked and bent in its own delicate, endearing misfittedness.

Michael has cerebral palsy, the spastic, hemiparetic form, which has left him with right-sided weakness and what we used to call mental retardation, or now, cognitive developmental delay. (Political correctness is a topic best left to another day.) Many people have varying degrees of cerebral palsy, some of which involve the entire body, but not the mind at all, others of which leave an individual profoundly limited, helpless, and dependent in all discernible aspects of life. Henri Nouwen describes such severely disabled people in his writings about the time he spent in the L'Arche community of Toronto.

Essentially, cerebral palsy is the result of what may be described as a stroke at birth. A physiologic stress right around the time of delivery leads to a lack of oxygen to the baby's brain, for various reasons and via various mechanisms. The pathophysiology is not what's important here. It is a moment of profound life-altering injury, much as any other serious injury occurring later in life might be. Part of the sadness is knowing how close the individual came to making it into this world as a whole and healthy person—just a little quicker, perhaps, into a gush of fresh air, into a nurse's cradling arms, a doctor's rescuing suctioning, just a saving moment and on to a "normal" life. But instead, they enter the world with a shriveled hand or with spastic bodies or with "brain damage." Too often now, such moments are legalized into lawsuits. There are no acts of God any longer. The anger and disappointment, grieving and loss must be vented somewhere, must have a target. The world is as we have made our dominion over it—give to Caesar what is Caesar's, to God what is God's, and give to me something to make up for my pain, my loss.

Quiet Suffering

We don't know why God allows such tragedies to occur. Why a lack of oxygen at birth, a near drowning at four, a spinal cord injury at nineteen, a head injury at twenty-five, an aneurysm at forty-seven, or a stroke just after retirement at sixty-five? People with such events in their lives can all look like my brother, can look like the man with the withered hand in the Gospel story, on the outside. What is the deeper image we are shown by this man, and even by the woman with her eighteen years of pain? It is their quiet suffering. It is their unassuming humility. It could be their weary brokenness, as in Iris's case, or it could be their gentle acceptance, as in my brother's.

My brother quietly, faithfully walks to church each day before he goes to his job. He may attend three or four Masses over the course of a weekend. People comment and are amazed at his humble reverence, his fervent look as he lights a candle and kneels before a statue of Jesus. They gaze into his bright, well-wishing eyes and his instant smile, even as they are caught off guard by the touch of his baby-soft, fragile-seeming hand as he says, "Peace be with you." He prays for others, for good weather, for his heroes: the firemen, paramedics, pilots, flight attendants, and air-traffic controllers. He prays for forgiveness when he feels he has done something wrong or said something hurtful to someone else. Such sweet, endearing humility. The man with a withered hand.

When he was a child, there were many times when we had to leave him behind with others, standing there crying, waving good-bye. As a young man, caught in childlike love of a pretty woman, he was crushed by circumstances that seemed to coldly reject him and blame him, and he cried to me in his grief on the phone. He stumbles and falls at times when he is in a rush to catch a bus, to be on time. Usually he bounces up. One time he broke his left arm—his good arm. He lay in the emergency room, frightened but courageous as the doctor checked him over. He was going to miss dinner, he thought, as he lay there waiting for a decision on surgery, and he was hungry. They cast his left arm, and I tried to imagine how he would do anything at all, since his poor little right hand was crippled already. I wrote on that day in my journal:

> Ah, my Lord, the young man cried his tears of anguish and outrage, question and confusion, frustration and helplessness. He stands truly almost helpless, right hand contorted, left hand now bound in the healing shell, evil though it appears, imprisoning, amputating almost . . . my worst nightmare. He cried, and I held him—neither of his arms able to embrace me back. I left him lying flat, still, with his arms and head propped on pillows in the bed. He likely felt he'd suddenly been laid in his dreaded coffin. I cry within and look to you. Bless him, dear Lord, that he may know that helplessness is not a sin, that asking for help is not failure, that receiving help is not humiliation. May my own faith be that of the centurion, who knew his own rushing and struggling were meaningless, and that his servant would be cured, if you but willed it so.

Another time, as he rushed to get ready for a first "date" that one of his counselors had arranged for him, he stumbled again on the sidewalk on his way to the bus. He completely scraped his face, lips, and arm on the right side. I was called and told that he was

being taken to the hospital. When I arrived, he was calmly waiting there. As I went to him, he stood up, reached his arms around
me, and began to sob uncontrollably. All the sadnesses of his life
seemed to flow from him as he stood within my embrace. All the
pains he quietly endured inside, all the things he perhaps wanted
that he couldn't have, all the prayers he offered that seemed to go
unanswered—he cried for it all in this eternal moment of broken-
heartedness. He didn't really hurt that much physically, as it turned
out, because all the scrapes were on his right side, which had less
acute sensation than his good, left side. His pain and sorrow were
deeper and were released in this instant of anguish. He had striven
for a happiness, a chance to have a date, a girlfriend like everyone
else, to be "normal" for a moment, and he was denied. As with
Jesus, he had stumbled again, under the weight of his cross. He
did not complain. He only cried. And he held out his wounded,
"withered" hand to the doctor.

Even now, he must bear up under another challenge. He fell
and broke his hip, landing awkwardly on his weak right side. Not
wanting to bother anyone, he did not call my parents until the next
morning. He stands up again, after this, his third fall along his own
Calvary road. Nervous and a little scared this time, he remains
cheerful and resilient. Onward, in innocence, he battles.

As for the man in the Gospel story made to stand in front of
everyone, we don't know the reason for his condition, nor do we
know what kind of man he was. I see him as sweet, endearing, and
humble—a man like my brother. He seemed to have just been there
in the synagogue that day, as my brother is so often in church, offering his simple prayers. Perhaps one of his prayers was in fact to be
healed of his shriveled hand. Or perhaps it was for a family member
who was ill or grieving. He could have been praying for a girl to like
him, who might accept him with his shriveled hand and one day
marry him. He might have been praying for the poor that he saw
around him or for a blind person he knew. He might have been there
because the Pharisees asked him, disingenuously, to come visit them

after Sabbath services, knowing him to be guileless and thus perfect for this trap they were trying to set for Jesus.

Brought Forward by Others

The bottom line is that the Gospel does not convey that this man brings himself before Jesus. He does not run up to Christ begging to be healed. He instead is brought forward, in front of this gawking crowd of Pharisees and onlookers. I see him a little fearful but trying to be polite and cooperative, because that is his nature. I envision him humble before the authorities of the synagogue and respectful before this stranger named Jesus, who seems to treat *him* with respect. As he is made to stand before the group, he is probably nervous and a little embarrassed, his small right hand perhaps wrapped in his stronger left. Yet he does not resist or question. He remains standing, the center of some kind of confrontation. Maybe he has seen Jesus around and knows him to be a kind man of special compassion and thus feels safe in his presence.

Even though the Gospel stories don't detail Christ's demeanor at this moment, we can infer from his beautiful mercy in the rest of the Gospels that he would act toward this gentle soul before him with the utmost kindness and care. He would emit a tremendous empathy toward him as he projects a calming assurance in this odd public arena. His gaze may reach this man's eyes, saying, "Trust in me. It will be all right. I will not let you be hurt." Let yourself feel Christ's infinite love in this scene, and thus you may begin to feel his infinite love for you in your own quiet moments of pain.

While the Pharisees don't really see a human being in front of them, but rather a prop, an object to further their own designs, Jesus sees one of his creatures in need of saving and protection. He sees each of us that way. In Matthew 12:12, Jesus points out how much more precious a human being is to God than property or animals are to their owners. Laws, social protocols, or concern for appearances or personal safety—all were put aside in service to the suffering people Jesus saw before him. He does not make these people earn their healing. It is a gift he gives. He wants to show how much love the Father has for us, and that God *will* intervene in our lives and rescue us.

In another passage, Jesus again takes the initiative:

> *As he drew near to the gate of the city, a man who had died was being carried out, the only son of his mother, and she was a widow. A large crowd from the city was with her. When the Lord saw her, he was moved with pity for her and said to her, "Do not weep." He stepped forward and touched the coffin; at this the bearers halted, and he said, "Young man, I tell you, arise!" The dead man sat up and began to speak, and Jesus gave him to his mother. (Luke 7:12–15)*

How God Finds the Lost

Each of the three stories presented here shows how God will find us, even when we are lost, even when we are too tired to call to him any longer and have given up. The poor woman bent over for eighteen years has lived with her affliction and, like the man with the shriveled hand, does not shout to Jesus to be healed. Perhaps they are both so humble and good-hearted that they accept their lots in life and strive to merely make it from one day to the next, never thinking to consider asking for more. We all know such quiet heroes; some of them are in our families. A mildly retarded nephew of a friend of mine was in the hospital with multiple complications of a complex combination of chronic disorders, yet while lying in bed in intensive care with tubes and IVs all over him, he genuinely beamed to his aunt and uncle, and exclaimed, "I've never felt better in my life!" There really are angels on this earth.

Others are spent and tired from the hardships of their daily struggles and do not have the energy to stand up boldly for themselves. Perhaps they feel unworthy to be asking for a miracle. They may feel guilty, shy, or afraid. They may even be too sad and despairing to hope that life could be different. It would be too crushing to be disappointed. Or they may be grieving the natural sadness that seems to occur randomly and sometimes cruelly, as in the case of the widow who has lost her only son.

They may be children, merely innocent, suffering, accepting the life granted them. They are humble. They are small, weak, and helpless. We fear for them and need to know that our God watches over them. It is so hard to let go of them to our God when we see them in pain or in danger.

Jesus steps into the lives of such innocents in the Gospels and lifts them up from their ordeals. It is hard to see this in our own lives sometimes, when tragedy and illness go on unchecked and unrelenting. The pure generous love of our God is present to those quietly bearing their pain. God sees the suffering and does something about it; it can be so difficult for us to see what this is, though, when looking into the eyes of a helpless child undergoing a bone marrow transplant, for instance, in the battle against leukemia.

God does not force us to beg for his healing. He does not blame us for our physical maladies. Though sin is acknowledged freely and frequently by Christ in the Gospels as a very real force in the world, he is adamant and clear about its lack of relation to people's diseases. The hallmark healing story confirming this is of the "man born blind," where Jesus is asked directly, "Rabbi, who sinned, this man or his parents, that he was born blind?" Jesus answered, "Neither he nor his parents sinned; it is so that the works of God might be made visible through him" (John 9:2–3).

In another location, while answering a question about a group who had been put to death by Pilate, Jesus is explicit in teaching his followers, and us, that our sins and our diseases are not cause-and-effect related.

> *He said to them in reply, "Do you think that because these Galileans suffered in this way they were greater sinners than all other Galileans? . . . Or those eighteen people who were killed when the tower at Siloam fell on them—do you think they were more guilty than everyone else who lived in Jerusalem?" (Luke 13: 2, 4)*

These are important messages to hear from our Creator, because no matter what we may say aloud, profess to believe, or intellectually accept, when we are suffering we cannot help wondering if we are being punished. Have we done something to deserve our pain? Have our sins come back to haunt us in this way? Or have we simply been too foolish or not careful enough? Because of our guilt, we often feel unworthy to turn to God for mercy. We feel that God is the one who has sent us our fates; therefore, how can we face him to ask for relief? The Gospel stories again demonstrate Jesus' desire to save us from our suffering. He shows that he will come to us wherever we are, even if we are too afraid, too guilty, or just too beaten to come to him. He says, "Come to me, all you who labor and are burdened, and I will give you rest. Take my yoke upon you and learn from me, for I am meek and humble of heart; and you will find rest for yourselves. For my yoke is easy, and my burden light" (Matthew 11:28–30).

Heroic Suffering

I have so many patients who are heroic in their suffering. Connie says, "I can handle the pain. Just give me some energy so I can do something with my life." Mildred tearfully asks for little, though she grieves the loss of her husband, endures the pain that persists in her back despite three operations, and worries over the struggles of a disconsolate son. Warren still laughs at my jokes, despite severe nerve pain from a back injury, the death of his son, the loss of his mother, and a stroke sustained by his wife. Harold grunts and struggles to move his spastic legs across the floor in his cerebral palsy, but he is gleeful at a small change I make to his brace. He leaves beaming on a snowy day, to take three buses home. Colleen remains faithful, cheerful, enthusiastic, forgiving, and ready to dance after five surgeries on a painful leg. Doug has been paralyzed for thirteen years and just wants to make sure the tiny movements remaining in his arms aren't lost, so he can keep himself independent and help his wife raise their family. His wife had been his nurse when he was first injured, and has given her life over to unconditional love.

Remember, the people in the Gospel stories who met Jesus and were "immediately" cured had often suffered patiently or hopelessly for many, many years. Even though you suffer now, you have no idea what is in store for you tomorrow. There are so many new technologies, procedures, medicines, and discoveries yet to be made that we cannot imagine what the future holds. Do not give up. Take advantage—realistically—of all that is available to get you through today. Balance this with acceptance, and you'll be prepared to fight through and survive whatever pain remains.

How does God let us know that he in fact sees us, cares for us, wants to stop an entire crowd in order to ask if we are all right? When we worry about our children or about the helpless disabled or elderly, the confused and lonely and poor, what assurance do we have that they will be cared for? Where among us is this Jesus, to protect those we love and to protect us when we are broken?

God needs *us* to step up and take action. He needs *us* to notice the weary and come to the hopeless, whether we know what to do for them or not. He needs the doctor to spend him- or herself by thinking a little harder, taking a little more time, and listening a little more closely. He needs the nurse to be a little gentler, a little quicker to answer the call button. He needs the therapist to be a little more creative, a little more willing to touch. He needs the priest to attend a little more as a true shepherd. He needs *someone* first to notice the shriveled hands, the stooped backs, and the silent grief. We need to come out of our lives and risk coming into the discomfort and pain of others. We need to acknowledge the neglected and to touch the rejected. We need to console the frightened and ask what it is we can do.

Whether it is another who is suffering or ourselves, someone needs to notice. Heed the constant call to be Christ for others. Be the miracle. Christ gently teaches us in his own words to "be compassionate even as your heavenly father is compassionate." God will find you, whether in the silence of your heart and mind, or through the gentle actions of those around you. Do not feel guilty when you are lying helpless in your suffering. Christ was pinioned helpless on the cross with and for you. Even when you are just too diseased, too much in pain, too tired to try anymore; even when it seems no one else cares or notices, remember that God sees you. God lifts your soul and touches your spirit. You cannot slip away from Him and His mercy.

Prayer of the Silent Suffering

Lord
You touched the leper, and he was healed
   Touch me.
You touched the blind man, and he could see
   Touch me.
You touched the bleeding woman, and she received your power
   Touch me.
You touched the children, and they laughed
   Touch me.
You touched the dead, and they lived
   Touch me.
Amen

Questions for Your Health

- Do you ever feel that you are being punished for something through your pain and suffering? Do you believe God would really do that to you? Does this feeling bring you closer to God or farther away?

- Most patients still respect their caregivers, doctors, and nurses. Nevertheless, do you give yourself permission to ask for more relief? Do you allow yourself the possibility of exploring other options elsewhere?

- Do you genuinely look for God's presence in your life through the actions of others, through the little turns of events that help you each day, mundane as they may be? Do you allow these little signs to assure you of God's working in your life? Try to notice at the end of each day how many small or large ways God has shown himself to you—in your thoughts, in the way circumstances worked out, in the kindness or talents of others.

- Turning that around, how many poor souls did you notice today who might have needed you to be God's relief for them?

9

"WHAT IS YOUR NAME?"

The Pain That Feels
Like Possession

O Lord . . . let my prayer come before you. . . . My soul is full of
troubles, and my life draws near to Sheol.

Psalm 88 (NRSV)

There are times when we are so lost in pain that we appear to
others possessed and unreachable. Our thrashing about, figuratively speaking (and at times probably not so figuratively), keeps
even those who used to be close to us at a wary distance. Our confusion, frustration, and pent-up sadness or rage can acquire such a
defensive edge that others don't want to be around us. Friends and
family tell us almost accusingly that we aren't the same as we used
to be, that we've changed into someone very unhappy. They try to
understand, but after a while they tire of focusing on our fluctuat-
ing tolerance levels. They seek to escape our oozing negativity. We
then watch from some isolated internal perch as the demons within
us run amock with our personalities, our sharpened tongues, and
our ugly behaviors.

Pain That Changes the Personality

At those times, we are caught in something very real and powerful. It is difficult to escape or pull out of our downward spirals, especially by ourselves. We do in many ways feel "possessed" by our pain and suffering. It has control of us, and we are no longer fully ourselves. We are too often distorted, surreal creatures of gloom and irritability. We hate what we are becoming, yet have little perceived capacity to break the hold of this power over us.

To a degree, we still expect sympathy and understanding. If those around us were forced to endure in their lives what we are being subjected to, they would be acting the same way. It's not really our fault. We feel unjustly abandoned when people start to drift away from us. We sink into pain that is more and more solitary. It is no wonder that this leaves us either depressed, with less energy for relationships and social interactions, or more irritable and thus less tolerable to be around.

It takes very committed friends and families to stick with us through these dark times. If these people are not strong, they may find it easier to just let us drift into a progressively more dysfunctional state. This is especially true if we respond to any intrusions by lashing back at those who seek to help us. They can be well-meaning and genuinely caring toward us, but we rebuff their efforts and cow them into throwing us scraps of sympathy from a safer distance.

To avoid confrontation, friends, family members, and caregivers may increasingly concede to our self-centered demands. By so doing, however, they inadvertently contribute to our decreasing sense of independence, and like adolescents we vacillate in a love–hate relationship with those whom we now need more than we want to admit. Our sense of personal responsibility starts to wane, and with it go our abilities to live in community with other adults. Should they attempt to go about their normal activities without us, we may react with a crisis of pain so disruptive that they have no choice but to attend to us, cancel plans, or bring us to the doctor or the emergency room.

Alan, Annihilated by Severe Pain

Alan's back had been injured playing sports a couple of years earlier, and he had been in increasing pain ever since. He was a nice guy with a great sense of humor, but the accumulating burden of pain was crushing him. He had quit his job and gone on disability; his wife was the main breadwinner now. Alan's pain medicines were his main solace. I would get calls that he was desperate, that he couldn't handle it anymore. We would talk things through and adjust his treatment.

But then his wife and brother would call, frantic that Alan was going crazy. I'd have them come in immediately. Alan would be writhing in agony, practically talking gibberish, looking like a shell-shocked prisoner of war, his face contorted tightly in a fit of crying. His helpless wife looked on in fear and disbelief as her husband grew less and less recognizable before her very eyes, lost in a psychological storm as much as in a physical illness. His brother tried to calm him down, while looking to me to do something, anything.

In these circumstances, we would put Alan in the hospital, alleviate his pain, and try to reorganize his life. It is amazing how dramatically the wailing and crying can cease, long before any medicine has had time to work, sometimes before the intravenous bottle has even been hung. So many patients and families who arrive at our offices ranting and nearly out of their minds are calmed by the mere knowledge that relief is possible and on its way. The groaning quiets and the tension eases.

Priscilla, Overwhelmed by Circumstances

Others wrestle longer with the devil, fighting off efforts to intervene on their behalf. Priscilla acted like a paranoid schizophrenic in her endless complaining about the thousands of things wrong in her life. When I tried to approach her problems one at a time, she could not get past the fact that there were too many problems, literally thousands ("My name is legion"). Her pains were every-where. They had been with her too long to be cured, yet she called me on Saturday and Sunday mornings, Friday nights, five times a day during office hours to decry her plight.

She made me think of a frantic bird trapped in a building, unable to alight on one spot long enough to be captured that she might then be set free. I finally told her she must speak directly to God if her problems were so great and so numerous. She was not allowing herself to be helped by mere mortals, for no matter what was offered her, she was sure it would never work because there was just too much wrong. It was sad not to be able to reach her.

A person can be so annihilated by chronic or severe pain, psy-chological suffering, or the emotional losses and upheavals of every-day life that he or she becomes a mere shadow of the former self. Many people have told me that I don't know them for who they really are, who they once were before all their problems and pain began. We all know people who for one reason or another have been altered by the years of physical or psychological turmoil. Many have fortresses of defense around them so intimidating that we dare not come too close for fear that we, too, may be sucked into their vortex of dysfunctional unhappiness.

In medicine, it takes effort to create the possibility of a miracle in such circumstances. It takes the interest and skills of caregivers to see through the barriers surrounding people in these situations in order to make a long-term difference in their lives. There is rage on the part of all involved whose lives have been altered by the power of pain. A chronic-pain unit in a hospital can sometimes look like the old images of insane asylums. And psychiatric units are filled with the pain of mental anguish and lost identities. People can be so "deformed" in their very personhood by suffering that they are unrecognizable for who they used to be. Caregivers and family mem-bers must pray to remain compassionate when patients and loved ones are no longer easy to care for and when they lash out in anger and despair rather than in gratitude.

It is hard to appear before others in our shattered states, after pain has had its long tyranny over us, and we no longer resemble who we thought we once were. Like the lepers, we cover ourselves in shame and cry out to others to stand back. Like the possessed, we sometimes fight and claw to resist anyone getting close because we hurt too much, physically, emotionally, and spiritually. God always steps through our personal storms to embrace us. Even screaming at God is at least contacting God. He can handle our pounding clenched fists, our accusations of betrayal and abandonment. God will not be intimidated. He can receive with love all the anguished whys sent over the centuries.

Is It All in Your Head?

"Doctor, are you saying that this is all in my head?" Well, in many ways, yes. All pain is, ultimately, a perception in the brain. This is simplified, to be sure. New thoughts on the neurophysiology of synapses and receptors at the level of the spinal cord, and also the quantum physics theories on holographic creative intelligence, have opened further questions about our entire understanding of "being," including being in pain.

If a patient with a spinal cord injury, paralyzed from the neck down, sustains a broken ankle, the fracture is not felt. There is no pain. On the other hand, we all have heard of phantom pain. An amputee feels his foot, even though he no longer has a foot. Where is that perception other than in his brain, where all the foot nerves terminate? Each of us has had the experience of the flashbulb that lingers in our vision after a photograph has been taken of us. Where is that image of a light still floating in front of us, except in our brains—not externally where the camera was. Hallucinations can be thought of in the same way. Thus, we must accept that pain as a perception, of even a very real injury or disease, ends up in our head.

This does not mean that pain is fabricated or that it is self-induced. Instead of getting caught up in whether, or how much of, your pain is "all in your head," can you at least consider that it is certainly "in your life"? And because it is in your life, can you recognize that it certainly affects many of the aspects of your life? Conversely, can you agree that the other aspects of your life—other events, stresses, emotions, and memories—can have at least a possible impact on the level of your pain and upon your ability to tolerate different levels of pain, at least on certain days?

The life in which your pain exists affects your pain, and that pain affects the life in which you live. True painful conditions or experiences, though very real in their sources of origin, must be seen to be experienced within the entire "universe" of the human brain. This includes those intangibles we label the mind, the psyche, the soul, and the personality. As such, all of these affect pain tolerance and pain behavior. In Ecclesiastes 3:11, it is said that God has placed eternity, or all that is timeless, into the human mind, or heart. Do not be so quick to recoil at the notion that pain is in your head—this is a big and powerful place, for harm but also for health, for hurting but for healing as well. With so much of the pain in our heads, how much of the healing is meant to occur in our heads also?

Jesus' Encounters with the Possessed

We become so afraid of pain's power. It is a demon to whom we have been given over for some reason, to whom the fates have allowed our lives to be sacrificed. If we dare reach out to be soothed, we are crushed by the devil of reprisal; hopes are dashed, and we feel brutally tossed aside for requesting any help at all.

Do we truly believe that God chooses to reach through all that makes us feel ugly? Jesus gently dismisses our storms, even as we cry out in ignorant fear. Look to the stories in the Gospels of those possessed.

These people were disconnected from intimacy and relationship by their unpredictable, unexplainable bizarre actions. Whether the people described were truly in some satanic state, or whether they instead suffered from psychological disorders, seizures, brain tumors, Huntington's disease, or any of a myriad of other mind-altering pathologies is not of great import here. Symbolically, they are images of us when we are frightened, trapped in our own hard-to-control anger, our own delirious states of pain and suffering, when the entire world seems to be our enemy.

As in almost all the healing stories, there is an engagement somehow between Christ and the sick person, even if brought about by someone else. Let us look at two of these particular encounters of Jesus, one with the Gerasene demoniac and the other with the possessed boy. In the former, a man (or two, as related in Matthew 8:28–34) brings himself to Jesus; whereas, in the latter, the boy is presented by his distraught father. So, too, we may drag ourselves before God, perhaps muddled by medicines and fatigue. Or, at other times, someone else seeks help for us, bringing the possibility of healing through their faith in what still may be possible. They may believe they have found the right expert, a unique doctor, or a special therapist, someone who will not waver before our intimidating defenses, someone who may have the gift necessary to exorcize our demons.

When he got out of the boat, at once a man from the tombs who had an unclean spirit met him. The man had been dwelling among the tombs, and no one could restrain him any longer, even with a chain. In fact, he had frequently been bound with shackles and chains, but the chains had been pulled apart by him and the shackles smashed, and no one was strong enough to subdue him. Night and day among the tombs and on the hillsides he was always crying out and bruising himself with stones. Catching sight of Jesus from a distance, he ran up and prostrated himself before him, crying out in a loud voice, "What have you to do with me, Jesus, Son of the Most High God? I adjure you by God, do not torment me!" (He had been saying to him, "Unclean spirit, come out of the man!") He asked him, "What is your name?" He replied, "Legion is my name. There are many of us." And he pleaded earnestly with him not to drive them away from that territory.

Now a large herd of swine was feeding there on the hillside. And they pleaded with him, "Send us into the swine. Let us enter them." And he let them, and the unclean spirits came out and entered the swine. The herd of about two thousand rushed down a steep bank into the sea, where they were drowned. (Mark 5:2–13)

Here is a raving maniac so frightening to those around him that he has been chained up. He is completely detached from society. Yet what does he do immediately upon seeing Jesus getting out of the boat? He *comes running up to him* and does him homage, not able to help crying out in a loud voice, so captive is he of his demons. Yet he fights the forces controlling him in order *to run toward Jesus rather than to run away from him.* The Gerasene demoniac practically launches himself toward Jesus, one part of him battling against all the rest, begging Jesus not to torment him.

Each of us can recognize similar moments, when we are caught between our love and our anger, toward others or toward God; handcuffed by our desires to be rescued and our resistance to that very need. Yet, if this man had never come running up to Jesus, he would not have been released from his demons. If he had not risked the encounter, even in his horribly messy condition, he would not have been made whole. Do you ever wonder how many other suffering people in Jesus' time never went up to him, and thus did not receive healing? Whether out of embarrassment, fear, humility, or some excuse, they did not overcome themselves or their demons in order to do what this man did.

The Courage to Move toward Jesus

People can become so hopeless and so identified with their illnesses that it is hard to convince them to try again. They have been betrayed too many times by those who were promising help. They feel worse every time they get up the courage to try to be more active, to get off the medicines, or to go back to work. It is only with the perseverance, commitment, and faith of all involved that such people can be given the tools with which to get better. It is difficult in these circumstances for families to trust in the process of expelling the demons of chronic illness.

What does Jesus do in this story? We can picture Jesus standing calmly as this poor man races toward him from the tombs. Christ does not run or back off. He simply asks, "What is your name?" In those words we hear his love, respect, and compassion toward a person whom everyone else has written off and avoided.

The moment is so full of reconciliation and rescue. It is so devoid of judgment and punishment. Our Lord gave but a "word" and it was done. Again, our God has the power to overcome whatever it is that exists between the created and the Creator. Whether of our own making or the result of sheer misfortune, our being possessed by illness, pain, addiction, anger, or depression is no match for God's desire to show us that we are known by name. God calls us beyond that which distorts our very natures. Created in God's image, we are sought out by our Creator so that we might be more fully alive as we are meant to be.

The Son Possessed

Often enough, it is the family members and friends who must remain faithful to a patient through the long suffering, through all the changes that also have become part of their lives as a result of someone else's misfortune. Through their trust, energy, and perseverance they remain with a patient until help comes.

> *Someone from the crowd answered him, "Teacher, I have brought to you my son possessed by a mute spirit. Wherever it seizes him, it throws him down; he foams at the mouth, grinds his teeth,*

and becomes rigid. I asked your disciples to drive it out, but they were unable to do so." . . . [Jesus said], "Bring him to me." They brought the boy to him. And when he saw him, the spirit imme-diately threw the boy into convulsions. . . . [The father said], If you can do anything, have compassion on us and help us." Jesus said to him, " 'If you can!' Everything is possible to one who has faith." Then the boy's father cried out, "I do believe, help my unbelief!" Jesus, on seeing a crowd rapidly gathering, rebuked the unclean spirit and said to it, "Mute and deaf spirit, I command you: come out of him and never enter him again!" Shouting and throwing the boy into convulsions, it came out. He became like a corpse.... But Jesus took him by the hand, raised him, and he stood up. (Mark 9:17–27)

So beautiful are the exchanges between Christ and this father, in the midst of what was at that time believed to be demonic possession. A picture of classic epilepsy and seizures could not be more accu-rately described in a medical textbook. Yet Jesus is not acting here as a neurologist, giving some secret anticonvulsant medication, or as some New Age practitioner, passing on a mind–body technique for ridding oneself of seizures.

Jesus first listens to the man's story and then asks for the child to be brought to him. The man asks Jesus if there is anything he can do to "help us." The suffering involves more than just the sick child. This father and the rapidly gathering crowd have brought Jesus into their communal situation. Illness can assuredly bring isolation to the one lost in misery, but it almost always envelops a broader circle of family, friends, and community. Addictions—to alcohol, drugs, gambling—are especially difficult examples of this suffering that draws down entire families.

We can imagine the father's hesitancy when he asks if Jesus "can" do anything. It's not said disrespectfully, and we imagine Jesus suppressing a smile when he repeats, "If you can?" He sees clearly the boundaries placed around this man by his society, his experiences, even his religion. This father is taking a risk in front of everyone to imagine openly that Jesus can do something.

And the man is not daunted by Jesus' comment. He stays right with Jesus, immediately admitting, okay, I believe. Help me. I'm ready. We're in your hands. Tell me what I need to do. Help us. "I do believe; help my unbelief!"

The Leap into Our Fears

This exchange between the father and Jesus reminds me of another story, of Peter seeing Jesus walking on the water and asking if he can join Jesus. Jesus says yes, and Peter begins to walk on the waves but falters and begins to sink. Jesus grabs his hand and pulls him up.

Our energy gains momentum once we have leapt into, and hence through, our fears. God does not play games with our vulnerability. Once we have entered the moment of love and trust, God remains with us, even when we panic at what we have done, as did Peter leaping out onto the water to walk toward Jesus. God does not criticize, ridicule, or abandon us for our weakness.

The father of the possessed boy saw in Jesus compassion and strength before which he could risk standing and pleading his son's case. He did not give up when the apostles had failed to help, and he did not waver or argue self-righteously with Jesus about his own level of trust. He just kept going. He stayed connected with Jesus. He was open to whatever Jesus could teach him in order to gain the healing he sought for his son, and for himself, in his own recognized lack of trust. He kept his eyes and hopes fixed on Jesus, even after other good men, Jesus' disciples, had failed, even as the demon threw down his son, almost scornful of this father's persistent devotion. In the midst of fear, this man did not panic, but immediately threw his trust over to God.

The Final Shriek

There is another image in both these stories of the possessed: the last shriek and episode of convulsing elicited by the demons, as Christ comes to the ill person. Before we make any meaningful leap, or just as others bring us to moments of decision, we can experience such dread or resistance, perhaps a final doubt. The vulnerable patient, in the end, is alone in the leap he or she has to take. Included in this leap is the very first step of saying, "I will go along with this. I trust you, doctor, and I will try what you suggest."

The mere suggestion of changing pain medicines can evoke tremendous anguish, arguing, and plea bargaining. Near panic can ensue at the mention of exploring a return to work in the face of continued pain. Tremendous fear can intimidate the person trying to decide whether to go ahead with a high-risk surgery. Dread can fill the heart of one who faces the beginning of chemo and radiation therapy. Family members are in a tough predicament. They sit on the edges of their seats, caught between rescuing their loved ones and realizing that some sort of "exorcism" needs to take place in these moments. Everyone in the room, for whatever the particular circumstances of a specific case, is aware of the leap of faith being called for. "Trust" is required of everyone.

Take for example the familiar story of Helen Keller, who was born with multiple impairments, including blindness, deafness, and the inability to speak. Her parents were completely ill equipped to deal with her. Neither were they supported in any constructive way by the medical and social networks of their day. In trying not to add to their daughter's sufferings, they were helpless to do no more than concede to her disruptive behaviors. As with all things ugly or embarrassing, such as deformity or addiction problems, society often tries to muffle the problem, to avoid the confrontations.

I have seen so many patients allowed to fall into terribly dysfunctional states as the result of well-intentioned medical professionals who instead of healing ended up creating or fostering medical "cripples." Initially sympathetic families also may have contributed to the regression of their loved ones into near invalids. Attempting to resist their own anger, weariness, and detachment, families are often left with no other strategy but to concede to the easiest courses that provide relief for a patient's suffering. However, the combined actions by patient, family, and caregivers serve, over time, to shrink the available world in which the suffering individual can live. Eventually that world, much like Helen's, becomes its own realm of pain and the behaviors that either express pain or avoid it.

When Annie Sullivan entered Helen's life, Helen was a wild, filthy little girl who had absolutely no meaningful connection to her community. It was a long journey of teaching, fighting, and epiphany. Called the "miracle worker" in the subsequent descriptions of her, Annie was one of those special determined people who saw the potential and not the futility in a situation. She brought the practical gift of sign language—a gift from God as true and real as any mud and spittle Jesus placed on the blind man's eyes that he might see (Mark 8:22–25). She brought the work of miracle making in the commitment of one person willing to give herself fully in service to another.

Though God did not cure Helen's eyes, ears, or tongue, she did somehow gain the gifts of vision, listening, and communicating. She did still suffer her physical limitations, but she became a new person, delivered from her prison and able to express and receive love.

The miraculous ripple effect of one life, Annie's, dedicated to another, Helen's, is astounding when we think of how their lives have influenced millions of blind and deaf persons since. Generations of individuals have been inspired to lead lives of service in special education, in schools for the blind and deaf, and in technological development of amazing assistive devices. So much was born out of the efforts of two women struggling with each other in a small room. As our Lord was not driven off by the raving demoniacs in the Gospel stories, Annie was not driven off by Helen's fits of rage, resistance, and fear.

In these stories of the possessed, we see that unfortunate people are often rejected because they are hard to be around or because their situations are too draining. They know they are hard to love. They know their pain can be frightening to people who just don't want to be around such constant unpleasantness. As with the possessed of Bible stories, they feel left to roam the outskirts of life, avoided by most. They *expect* people to back away from them. After a while, they start to behave in self-fulfilling ways, and a vicious cycle is created.

In the world of pain and suffering, we can easily lose touch with our better selves. We can fight against the very goodness that seeks to help us. Let us pray to recognize the miracles as they come to us from God, who may send us our own Annie Sullivans, to drag us, kicking and screaming, through our fears, until we finally receive deliverance. With compassion and power, Christ reminds us to trust. In the face of whatever ugliness we feel we bring, he commands the demons in us to be gone and frees us to leave the tombs, to reenter our true lives.

Run to Me, Your God

Do you believe you have in you a spirit too evil to be helped by God?
Do you feel anger and coldness toward God?
Do you feel too far gone to ever be forgiven?

As the poor demoniacs, running amock amid the tombs,
You too may be rejected by those around you, avoided, forgotten.
But I, the Lord, still loved these raging men whom society could not understand.
How could I not love you, one of my very own, for all the wonder of you, bottled up inside?
Run to me. Do not stay away. Do not hide.
All others may keep their distances out of fear or frustration.
But I cannot be any closer than I already am.

Your soul will be drawn to me, even when your anger hates me or
your confusion has you lost.
Love will overcome.
I will recognize you when you yourself have already forgotten who
you are.
I will ask your name.
I will break your chains.
I will set you free.

Questions for Your Health

- Illness can so dominate us that our identities are almost more medical than personal. In what ways has your pain or your condition made the real you invisible? What is the most meaningful part of you that most others have not been able to see or know about you?

- How might you become less known for your headaches, your back pain, or your heart condition and more known for your intelligence, sense of humor, kindness, or even your selfless perseverance?

- Has going to confession ever crossed your mind—not to cure your illness, but to soothe your soul? Have you been open to seeing a counselor or psychologist to unburden you of the isolation you've suffered because of your illness? If not, why not? God may be just waiting to talk to you somewhere, while you keep yourself holed up in your house, too embarrassed and ashamed at the depths to which you have sunk.

- As parent or spouse of someone in need of God's touch, do not grow weary of seeking help. Remember that in the Gospel story the apostles had already tried and failed to help the father and his son. The father did not give up and finally found the right person in Jesus. In medicine, good doctors and therapists will know other good doctors and therapists. Start with who you know and work your way to who you need.

10

"WERE NOT ALL TEN CURED? WHERE ARE THE OTHER NINE?"

The Healing Work of Gratitude

Be gracious to me, O Lord, for I am in distress. . . . For my life is spent with sorrow, and my years with signing; my strength fails because of my misery.

Psalm 31 (NRSV)

A patient came in with her parents, though she was in her late twenties. She was shaking, sweating, constantly shifting her position around the room. She used a cane to get around, and she grunted and groaned with each effort. She looked ready to fall or pass out with every movement. Her parents did most of the speaking for her, so distracted was she by her condition.

She cast a wary look at me, the next new doctor. She'd worn down many a specialist before. She undoubtedly anticipated that this relationship wouldn't last long and, like prior relationships with doctors, wouldn't benefit her much.

She was consuming a tremendous amount of pain medicines but not really gaining relief from them. At this point, she'd taken so many that she was in a state of physiologic tolerance. Her metabolism was getting rid of the narcotics so efficiently that she was in constant pain from too little analgesic, combined with a state of true withdrawal. She bore the haunted, restless appearance of a drug addict.

Another patient came in by wheelchair because he had been in too much pain to walk for the previous eight months. Nevertheless, he was calm, talkative to the point of being glib, and amazingly not at all disturbed at his level of illness. He reported not only back pain but also memory problems, headaches, a progressively weak ankle, sexual difficulties, an inability to spend any time with his two children, and a need to remain in bed nearly twenty hours a day. He was taking forty-five different pills daily for his various maladies.

He had a fairly normal exam, other than a lot of grimacing when he had to get out of the wheelchair and get up on the examining table. His neurologic and orthopedic functions were in order, but he said it was very difficult for him to move around. He was thirty-six and had come on his own from a great distance.

The first patient had endured three spine surgeries, with the initial one resulting in a severe infection, thus necessitating a subsequent emergency operation, followed finally by a third, which involved a large fusion procedure. She was in horrible pain and was exhibiting signs of nerve damage. She was psychologically broken. In addition, she was now terribly overweight from her inactivity and her overeating, a response to her empty life and growing depression. The first treatment priority was to develop for her a more effective regimen of pain relief while assisting her out of her entanglement of narcotic dependency. This would require a great amount of willpower on her part, as it seemed to her that she was already not receiving enough pain medicine. She was also given a plan of rehabilitation for her weakness, walking difficulties, spine instability, and overall deconditioned state.

The second patient had had only a minor motor-vehicle accident two years earlier. He had had a history of several work injuries before that. None of his tests had shown any signs of damage to his nerves, discs, bones, or muscles. Yet over the two years since his accident, one part of his physiology after another had apparently and mysteriously become dysfunctional, though none of the doctors could quite figure out why. It just seemed that the accident had caused a disruption in his entire life. All the MRIs and scans were negative, and every therapeutic measure made him feel worse. His life was completely on hold, with no medical end in sight.

Two Different Responses

The first patient followed the plan provided her, struggled mightily with her pain while sincerely making a good effort at decreasing her medications. She remained faithful to her therapy schedule, and conveyed that she felt she was actually making some progress. At this point, she took a sudden turn for the worse, as far as her overall health was concerned, and was hospitalized in intensive care. Through a comprehensive set of evaluations, she was found to have a liver disorder, which had weakened her system, but was fortunate to have it successfully managed and fully resolved. She couldn't believe the new energy she felt. She sensed she had been given a new lease on life, and that she now had an explanation for at least part of why she had felt so lethargic and so ill over the past year. She had thought it was all due to her spine surgeries. The new findings helped her understand, too, why she might have been susceptible to an infection from her surgery in the first place.

She enthusiastically pushed to accelerate her rehabilitation, as well as the tapering off of her pain medicines. She admitted that she was still in pain but that she felt better, more energetic and clearheaded, and more in control of her life since freeing herself from all the drugs she had been taking before. She was thrilled that she was losing weight and getting into better physical condition. She wanted permission to join a health club and to work out on her own. She also was making plans to get some further schooling so she could qualify for a job position she had discovered. She returned to tell me how well she was doing.

The second patient was also given rehabilitation options, a medication reduction plan, and an outline for regaining some of the value and productivity in his life, perhaps allowing him to be able to participate as a parent to his children again, and to put back into his future some hope of a more normal life. As it turns out, though, he had already filed for full disability and was waiting for that to come through. In addition, he had a lawsuit pending in his automobile accident case and was claiming complete incapacitation as a result. He very pleasantly anticipated that he would be spending the rest of his life at leisure, and he seemed quite content with his low state of functioning. And off he went.

> As he continued his journey to Jerusalem, he traveled through Samaria and Galilee. As he was entering a village, ten lepers met [him]. They stood at a distance from him and raised their voice, saying, "Jesus, Master! Have pity on us!" And when he saw them, he said, "Go show yourselves to the priests." As they were going they were cleansed. And one of them, realizing he had been healed, returned, glorifying God in a loud voice; and he fell at the feet of Jesus and thanked him. He was a Samaritan. Jesus said in reply, "Ten were cleansed, were they not? Where are the other nine? Has none but this foreigner returned to give thanks to God?" Then he said to him, "Stand up and go; your faith has saved you." (Luke 17:11–19)

There are some people whom God himself, coming down from heaven, could not cure. They are just not open to the offer. God *did* come down from heaven on high and cure the lepers. Yet they didn't know the difference, didn't recognize the cure, and wouldn't accept the miracle. They might have been so "into" being lepers, might have been so identified with their disease at that point in their lives, that they were blind to the fact that the disease itself was suddenly gone—that God had actually heard them and healed their pain!

Sometimes people are not ready for such a change in their lives. They feel safer right where they are. They can block even divine efforts, quite persistently. "Thank you, Lord, really. That was so very kind of you to try, but this problem is so much more difficult than everyone else's. You know, I've just resigned myself to living with it. The doctors try to help, and so does my family. I do whatever they ask me to, but nothing ever works. Again, thank you anyway." And off they go down the lanes, continuing to keep their distance and lamenting their leprosy.

To this day, God comes down from heaven on high, so to speak, to offer us all sorts of cures and balms for that which ails us. But we can resist. We can be blind. All the most modern technological advances in microinvasive procedures and devices can be brought to bear, with no effect. The best medicines can prove powerless: "Well, they all just make me groggy, Doctor, or they just don't work. I react to all of them." All of them? Every pain-blocking injection? Every single one, of all different classes of chemical structure and type? "They all made me worse, Doctor." Even while the anesthetic was numbing the tissue? That was a lot of numbing medicine. "Oh, that stuff never works on me, Doctor." Surgeries? "They didn't do a thing for me, Doctor. It's like I never even had anything done. I'm exactly the same." All the doctor's time spent listening, explaining, teaching, and consulting leads nowhere. "No one understands. I mean this pain is bad. You just don't know." What about alternative and complementary options? "Nope, Doc, I tried all that stuff. Doesn't do anything."

To be sure, there are many cases where true pain remains despite the best efforts of patients and their treating teams. The point is not so much one of technicalities and outcomes, but of attitude and participation.

The Instinct for Keeping Distance

What is the difference between these ten lepers and the other lepers cured in the Gospels? The ten lepers kept their distance from Jesus. We know this was a cultural code of behavior that was expected of lepers at the time of Jesus, yet in the Gospels these were the only ones who kept their distance from him. The leper early in the Gospels came right up to Jesus and asked to be cured. Others were brought to him, and he laid hands upon them. As we have just seen in the previous chapter, even the possessed demoniacs ran up to him.

An intimacy needs to exist between the sick person and the miracle worker. There are patients (and doctors, too, for that matter), however, who do not engage well in the therapeutic encounter. There exists a distance separating these patients from those trying to help them, even in the confines of a doctor's tiny office. Such is the feeling one gets from patients who seem to be resisting care or who never seem satisfied, or who can never admit that they feel even a little better. They may have already made up their minds about who they are going to be and how they are going to live the rest of their lives, much like the second man described in the patient stories above.

The Gospel account says of the lepers, "They raised their voices." Sometimes patients feel unheard in trying to convey their exact pains to the doctor. "Doctor, I don't think you understand what it is I am going through! My pain is never just a ten out of ten. It is a thirteen on the good days and goes up to a twenty when it really gets bad!"

I have to say that sometimes it's not the patient who is responsible for the lack of true engagement. There are too many health-care experiences today in which it is in fact the doctors or nurses or other health-care professionals who are not listening to, not hearing the cries of their patients. Sometimes doctors are so cold, impersonal, rushed, or lacking in compassion, that they almost force patients and families to "raise their voices" in order to be heard.

A friend shared with me a horrendous experience he had with a loved one's course of illness and care in a hospital. His family member eventually died. This family was in the hospital every day to give support. In asking for information or advice, they felt so unheeded that they became almost like this roving band of lepers, ostracized even by those who were supposed to help them the most. There are many examples in the Gospels where Christ reserved his worst admonitions for those who were supposed to be the healers: the Pharisees, the priests, even his own disciples. Thus, I don't want the reader to feel that the onus is always on the patient. It is for the point of this chapter, however, that I look at patients who have become too mired in their own plights, regardless of the skills and attitudes of their doctors.

Perhaps as with the lepers, such patients have just grown used to lamenting their plights loudly for all to hear. They can't tell you enough how much they are hurting and how no one cares. They are deaf within their own pain zones. They hear no solutions; they hear no answers to their prayers; they hear no voice of God. There are also those who do not trust being near others, and they behave in ways that keep distance between themselves and others, between themselves and love.

What did the lepers specifically ask of Jesus? To be cured? No, they cried, "Have pity on us!" Surely others in the Gospels asked for Jesus' pity, but in this story, with the exclamation point, these lepers weren't so much asking for the Lord's pity as they were demanding it. Patients will demand, "Do something! I shouldn't have to live like this! I am too young to be dealing with this. I can't play golf. I can't live with this disorder for the rest of my life!" Rather than expressing an interest in being healed, some convey a sense of entitlement. Their lives should be instantly freed of the inconveniences unfairly foisted upon them.

Others just flounder in wailing and complaining. Their words, "Have pity on us," are almost mantras of habit, chanted now without genuine desire or true searching. They don't look for the rope tossed to them. They don't hear the words of advice. They are busy thrashing—not truly panicking, just thrashing. Getting healthier is not necessarily on their agendas. For them, nothing changes when relief is offered. It's almost as if they interpret any offer of help as an effort to suppress them and make them go away.

Risks of Getting Better

Do we, as friends, family, and caregivers, sometimes make it hard for people to become better? Do some individuals get more love and attention, care and company, from being sick than they ever received from us when they were healthy? Do some lonely people find that coming to the doctor provides the social attention and acknowledgment otherwise absent in their lives? Where would all the concern and sympathy go if suddenly they were no longer sick? Would friends and family disappear back into their own busy lives? Would the doctor say, "Great, you don't need to come back anymore," and dash out the door? What if patients feel fragile and afraid of being left on their own? What if they get thrown back into the cold pit of work where no one cares how they feel? What if their families expect them to just pick up where they left off, get back to making dinner, running errands, picking up the kids, going out to uncomfortable business dinner parties, even going on long vacations? Normal life can be quite daunting to the person who has been sick a long time. Getting better, strangely, seems scary.

We can get too comfortable with the lowered expectations that result from long illness. We have built up so many walls to protect ourselves that we've become quite isolated. Giving up the few people tied to us by our sickness will leave us frighteningly on our own. Better to not admit the medicine is working or that the injection actually helped. "I think I still need the physical therapist to work with me." Locked in such a state, we allow no room for true gratitude to others or even to God. We are afraid to give even that little part of ourselves that lets another person know that what they are giving to us is actually helping, because we dread that when they perceive that we don't need them anymore, they'll abandon us. Ironically, after a while our caregivers may give up on us anyway, weary of negative results and no positive feedback.

Although others may leave us, God never will. Jesus did hear from afar the cries of this roving band of lepers. He recognized their loneliness and their disconnection from society, and he sent them back to reconnect: "Go and show yourselves to the priests." He sent them from where they stood. He didn't ask them to do anything but perhaps *change the direction in which they were walking*. But oh how hard it can be for us frail creatures of habit to make changes in our lives, even when, in truth, we hate where we are.

The story does not say that the nine lepers *never* came to recognize themselves as being cured. For some, it might have taken years to overcome an identity that had been so scarring. It might have taken a slow series of risks to gain the courage to step back into a society that had rejected them and treated them cruelly. God can wait. He seeks the lost lamb, even after the ninety-nine have long ago been found. God has the time. We are the only ones who can waste that precious gift.

Caregivers as well as families need to be patient, as do sick people themselves. Jesus does challenge us sometimes, even while he heeds our loud cries. The answers to our prayers may not come in packages we expect. Not every pain or problem will disappear just because we cooperate with a medical plan, work hard in rehabilitation, or say some prayers. Are we open to accepting as our daily bread whatever God chooses to provide this day?

The Contribution of Gratitude

As for the principle of gratitude itself, we cannot be grateful for what we do not recognize. Do we see the nearness of our God? Are we ready to get beyond our demands for pity? Will we express gratitude for the efforts of others to remain with us, for the efforts of those trying to help us? This turning outward in gratitude, in spite of the pain that remains, may allow for God to reveal to us a new way through our problems. He may send us to "show" ourselves to the priests, so to speak, to someone who may have solutions for our conditions.

The one leper realizes right away the gift he has received and returns to Jesus in gratitude. He comes to Jesus in this new mind-set, where before he had kept his distance. He returns to Jesus perhaps less afraid to be intimate. He is no longer an outcast. The key is that he recognizes this, accepts his new freedom, and acts out of his new identity.

Gratitude for even little things brings us into closer touch with others and with our God. Gratitude is a sharing, an acknowledgment to someone else that we have received something from them. By its nature, it bonds us to one another. As a state of mind and an attitude of the heart, it brings us closer to God.

Focusing beyond terrible circumstances allows us to see. If we cannot see, we cannot recognize a gift. Without this openness, vision, and recognition, we express no gratitude. We do not fully connect then with those giving of themselves to us. There is no growth of intimacy. Rather, we continue down the road, lonely and lamenting loudly. We don't see that it is Jesus standing right before us, hearing our cries, and answering us. We do not see God working a miracle in us.

Pray for your caregivers to have the patience and perseverance to stick with you while you heal. Pray for yourself to have the courage to overcome your fears of change. Be patient with those, or with yourself, who have become disillusioned as a result of long suffering. It takes some people longer than others to see and to believe that they have been cured. But God does not disappear or walk away.

The Gospels show us how simply Christ offers a new lease on life, with the words, "Go and show yourselves to the priests." Jesus was there when the one leper came running back to him in gratitude. God happily awaits your returning to him in thanks. He wants to give so much more. He often gives us one step at a time so that at each point along the way we can grow into a deeper awareness of the fullness of his love. We are blessed then with the vision to see more and more all the gifts he places around us each day. By living in a state of gratitude, we are granted solace by all the graces we then see in our lives, and we are less caught up in a lonely travail of endless, wandering sadness.

The Lord Longs to Give—Be Open to Receive

Ah, weary ones, so lost in your sadness and grief.
You do not even see the Lord walking toward you.
You do not hear His gentle voice asking how He can help.
You do not even feel His touch as He seeks to embrace you.

The Lord will cure you anyway, in your heart,
And He will remain with you until you know in your heart that He
*   is there.*
He will always be there,
No matter your lament, no matter the distance you try to keep.

Questions for Your Health

- How would you assess the quality of the communication you have with your doctor? Focus more on the level of understanding between the two of you. Do you feel that you are heard?

- How do you think your doctor would describe your ability to listen and be open to what he or she suggests?

- List three ways your situation has already improved since you started treatment for whatever it was that brought you to the doctor or therapist. Decide each day to be grateful for some aspect of your healing. The magic is that the more grateful you choose to be, the more healing you will become aware of and, likely, the better you will feel, even if on the surface your condition does not seem to go away.

- Are there ways you find you tend to hold onto your illness and thus keep your distance from others? If so, why do you think this is? Pray to recognize how much God has already healed you, and ask how you may be of service to someone else.

11

"HE COULD WORK
NO MIRACLES THERE."

The Sin of Resistance

*How long, O Lord? Will you hide yourself forever? How long will your
wrath burn like fire? Remember how short my time is. . . . Who can
live and never see death?*

Psalm 89 (NRSV)

There is a rarer, but more sinister, type of patient, which I hate
to even bring up, yet our Lord speaks directly to it himself. It is
the patient who brings a true hardness of heart into the therapeutic
encounter. Not all are willing to be reconciled. And each of us carries the capacity for sin.

The parable told by Christ in Matthew 22:1–14 and in Luke
15:16–24 conveys an intriguing image of what the reign of God can
be likened to. In this story, a king gives a wedding banquet for his
son, and all the invited guests turn him down. Some of them even
kill the messengers. So the king sends his servants into the streets
to bring in all the poor, the lame, the beggars, and so on, in order
to fill his banquet hall. He commands that anyone—good, bad, or
otherwise—is to be invited.

But there is one poor fellow who shows up at the feast not properly
dressed for a wedding. It seems to me that this man shows up just as he's
always been, a poor beggar perhaps. He hasn't crashed the party or tried

to sneak in. Someone came up to him on the street and invited him to the king's home for this feast. Is he given leeway? Let's read on:

> *"But when the king came in to meet the guests he saw a man there not dressed in a wedding garment. He said to him, 'My friend, how is it that you came in here without a wedding garment?' But he was reduced to silence. Then the king said to his attendants, 'Bind his hands and feet, and cast him into the darkness outside, where there will be wailing and grinding of teeth.' Many are invited, but few are chosen." (Matthew 22:11–14)*

Originally that seemed a little harsh; then it dawned on me. The king generously offered to lavish his goods upon people with whom he had no connection whatsoever. All were invited, the bad as well as the good. It doesn't say whether this man was specifically poor, lame, or immoral. Obviously, Christ is speaking through a parable, and thus we are not meant to take its components literally.

What may matter is how this man brought himself to the encounter, how he responded to the invitation. Does he recognize that he is being offered a gift? Does he bring himself to the moment in gratitude, in respect, and with his best foot forward? When given the opportunity to explain himself, "he was reduced to silence." He is seemingly too self-absorbed to perceive God inviting him to join the great party. This is so different from the woman bent over or the man with the withered hand. Though they had most probably been going about their painful existences for years, quietly and unobtrusively, each "immediately" received the cure offered when Jesus brought them into the "party" and called them to stand up front.

The Reality of Evil

In the Gospels, the existence of evil is unquestioned. There are evil people, evil circumstances, and evil forces. Christ makes it clear that life presents choices and that behaviors have consequences. He is also clear that he chooses to love, forgive, and accept us. Our actions, behaviors, and responses, however, direct the outcomes of our encounters with him. The parable of the seed sown on poor soil versus good soil is just one example of Jesus explaining that not all will accept his offer of love. The parables of the vineyard owners, the kings, and the masters in relation to their servants and hired hands demonstrate how some people are good and some are bad.

Christ does not hesitate to include in those stories the "wrath" of the angered or disappointed owners and kings generated by the evil actions of their subjects or servants. He does not wince in describing punishments. This is a little scary to read when we've let ourselves off the hook for a lot of our own failings, failings we have excused as just so much acceptable imperfection in our natures. We have told ourselves that God doesn't really expect perfection from us anyway. We have chosen to hear the soft words from a tolerant parent and have turned deaf ears to the tougher words of a just disciplinarian. We have for the most part dismissed the possibility that God would ever be so harsh as to send us to hell for all eternity.

Jesus names the sinfulness in the world and acknowledges that people must deal with evil. Through the story of the wheat and the weeds, he states that both will be allowed to grow together until they are separated at the harvest. Meantime, in order to protect the good, the bad will not be weeded out. This implies that this mix of good and bad is sown into our hearts. We would be destroyed if the freedoms granted us by the Creator were manipulated in order to eliminate evil. We must live and grow, struggling along the way.

Christ does not discount the presence of evil in the world and its ability to cause suffering now and spiritual consequences in the future. There is in fact one thing that can block Jesus' ability to perform miracles. That is the hardness of our hearts.

The Gospels report that throngs of people came to Jesus and were healed. And there are two accounts of Jesus miraculously feeding crowds with a few loaves and fishes. It is evident that thousands of people experienced firsthand the healing power of Christ. All their illnesses were cured; even the dead were raised. How could Christ be doubted? We may find it incredible that in the face of such wonders, some still resisted believing in the divinity of Jesus.

Jesus was patient with those who had difficulty accepting him out of fear, uncertainty, or an inability to understand. With those people, he gave further explanation or further challenge. But he could not rescue those who came with utter certainty of their lack of faith in him, with absolute self-righteousness and arrogance in their disputes against him. Their own walled hearts sealed out even the power of God's love. They had the same opportunity and access as anyone else, but they refused it. While some became able to see, hear, walk, speak, and breathe because of Jesus, others became frenzied in an effort to snuff him out.

Some people had already made up their minds about Jesus. And their opinions and beliefs didn't budge, even in the face of all the reports about him, even when they, themselves, witnessed his power.

> He came to his native place and taught the people in their synagogue. . . . And they took offense at him. But Jesus said to them, "A prophet is not without honor except in his native place and in his own house." And he did not work many mighty deeds there because of their lack of faith. (Matthew 13:54, 57–58)

In Mark the same story concludes this way:

> So he was not able to perform any mighty deed there, apart from curing a few sick people by laying his hands on them. He was amazed at their lack of faith. (Mark 6:5–6)

And even in those towns where miracles had been performed, many were not satisfied or convinced enough to follow what Jesus taught on how to live:

Then he began to reproach the towns where most of his mighty deeds had been done, since they had not repented. . . .

For if the mighty deeds done in your midst had been done in Sodom, it would have remained until this day. But I tell you, it will be more tolerable for the land of Sodom on the day of judgment than for you. (Matthew 11:20, 23–24)

Despite the multiple marvels surrounding Jesus, many just weren't satisfied. "'Teacher, we wish to see a sign.' He said to them in reply, 'An evil and unfaithful generation seeks a sign.'" (Matthew 12:38–39).

One of the more popular Gospel stories is the raising of Lazarus, in John chapter 11. A great many people are present when Jesus calls a man from the tomb in which he's lain dead at least four days. It's obvious to us now that a great miraculous event was taking place. Of course we would have believed in him if *we* had been standing there watching. Yet, somehow, real people just like us were standing there, and even after witnessing for themselves the dramatic raising of a person from the dead, before throngs of other witnesses, they refused to allow for a personal change of heart about this enemy Jesus, so hardened were they against him:

But some of them went to the Pharisees and told them what Jesus had done. So the chief priests and the Pharisees convened the Sanhedrin and said, "What are we going to do? This man is performing many signs. If we leave him alone all will believe in him, and the Romans will come and take away both our land and our nation." . . . So from that day on they planned to kill him. (John 11:46–48, 53)

Let's say we didn't like anything about this Jesus and suspected he was a manipulator and deceiver, even if we couldn't figure out how he was pulling it off. Everything he did enraged us, especially as we saw more and more people running after him, beguiled, misled, caught up in the excitement. This is how we often react toward our political leaders. It is also how we sometimes act in response to family, friends, or doctors who seek to tell or show us what we don't want to hear or see.

It is difficult to acknowledge our own complicity in that which ails us. This can include dissatisfaction with a job or a relationship. It can relate to being overweight or being unhealthy in habits such as smoking or drinking. It can center around allowing ourselves to become totally inactive or depressed in response to pain or disease. When others even dare suggest that perhaps there are things we could do to help ourselves, we harden. When we are offered options that we have always considered foolish or beneath us, we harden. When it is implied we must go on in spite of the imperfections in our lives, we harden.

The apostles themselves responded with bewilderment to Jesus' discourse on eating his body and drinking his blood: "This saying is hard; who can accept it?" Jesus asks, "Does this shock you?" (John 6:60–61). He has no problem engaging us right where we are, if we at least open ourselves to be engaged. Doubt and frustration are not sins. The wrong occurs when we close our hearts and minds. "As a result of this, many [of] his disciples returned to their former way of life and no longer accompanied him" (John 6:66).

But Peter speaks for the faithful, if as yet still lost and uncertain, when Jesus asks the twelve if they, too, are going to leave. "Master, to whom shall we go? You have the words of eternal life" (John 6:68). The tone seems to be sad yet devoted. The apostles are struggling with all that surrounds Jesus and his teachings; yet they hang on, because they accept in him a power greater than themselves. This humility is what gets them beyond their own doubts or fears. Many times we are called to remain faithful to God, even when it seems the hardships we are forced to endure will be all too much for us.

But when we harden our hearts, we refuse to consider that there is power beyond ourselves. We become blind to what is right in front of us. We simply refuse to be changed or to follow someone's lead.

Hardness of heart develops when our personal agendas outweigh any evidence to the contrary.

> *"Why do you not understand what I am saying? Because you cannot bear to hear my word. You belong to your father the devil and you willingly carry out your father's desires. . . . there is no truth in him. . . . But because I speak the truth, you do not believe me. Can any of you charge me with sin? If I am telling the truth, why do you not believe me? Whoever belongs to God hears the words of God; for this reason you do not listen, because you do not belong to God." (John 8:43–47)*

Jesus is quite direct in his criticism of evil, pride, and a hardened lack of faith. In Matthew 23, Jesus utters a vitriolic tirade against the evil he has found in some men's attitudes and actions, especially in how this evil affects and brings down others. "Woe to you, scribes and Pharisees, you hypocrites." (Matthew 23:13). In various translations he calls them "blind guides," "hypocrites," "blind fools," "full of filth and dead bones," "whited sepulchers," "murderers," "vipers' nest," "brood of serpents." This is the loving, forgiving, compassionate, gentle Jesus in whom we put all our trust, who will show us mercy and forgive us our little failures and indiscretions!

In the Gospels, there were those who were too arrogant to see themselves as broken, sick, or sinful. Therefore, they had no use for Jesus. Not only were they blinded to their own imperfections, they also were enraged and angered that others chose to heed Christ's words. They would not be open to new ways of looking at the world or at themselves. Jesus threatened the status quo and challenged their deep-seated ways of thinking. He was inviting them out of their comfort zones, to risk seeing in a new way. This was too much for them to bear. They lashed out at it and tried to make it disappear.

> *For everyone who does wicked things hates the light and does not come toward the light, so that his works might not be exposed. (John 3:20)*

A Medical Version of Hard-Heartedness

The presumption in the world of doctor–patient relationships is that each person is being honest and genuine with the other. It would seem to go without saying that all patients truly desire to be cured, and that all physicians and other caregivers are sincerely trying their best to provide a cure. Yet this is not always the case. There are those few times when a physician walks into a room and senses in the presence of the patient or an accompanying family member what can only be called evil. (Patients have probably felt the same about some doctors they have faced.) Here is one such patient I encountered.

In the work-injury clinic, it was my job to take care of the patients medically, while judging as fairly as I could whether they could work in some capacity. It was always a negotiation. Some people were more straightforward in their demeanors: "Just wrap me up so I can get back to the line, Doc." Others were manipulative: "Aw, c'mon, Doc. My back is killing me. *You* don't have to bend over all day. It's Thursday—can't you just give me off till Monday? I start my vacation that day, and I'll be off for two more weeks. It'll help me get better faster."

On a particularly busy day of one patient after another, I was brought up short by a man whose very body language conveyed something ominous. There was hardness to his facial expression so implacable as to be threatening. Neither of us had spoken a word, but the room seemed filled with evil.

This man was dressed in what appeared to be expensive, chic clothing. He had on sleek gloves, a velvet scarf, a leather jacket, a matching sweater with turtleneck underneath, tailor-fit pants, and designer boots. He wore a stylish hat and sunglasses, though the lights in the clinic were not that bright. He didn't move from his slouched position on the chair and barely grunted when he responded to my questions. My job, obviously, was to sign a piece of paper that would maintain his no-work status. He said he couldn't do anything with his hands because of their pain. There was nothing at all he could do with his hands that would allow him to work, not even walking around the warehouse looking at tally sheets or monitoring safety compliance.

In my attempts to interact with him, I could tell that any energy he spent responding to me was given grudgingly at best. I decided to risk testing him a little, before trying to make a conclusion about him one way or the other. I acknowledged how finely his multiple layers of clothing matched, and asked if his hands hurt when he got himself dressed. He said sullenly that his wife helped him. I then asked more specifically if she put on his shoes for him, his socks, his gloves, his pullover sweater and turtleneck. He said yes, his wife did all that. No offense, but did she button his shirts and help him with his underwear, too? He had said he was 100 percent unable to use his hands in even the slightest way that would allow him to work. Did she cut up his food, spoon- and fork-feed him, because he couldn't hold a utensil at all? "Yep," is all he muttered, with deepening disgust for me, not once moving an inch from the posture he had when I entered the room. I went on a little more, then ceased, realizing how much the room was filled with a deadness of spirit. Negative energy can be palpable, its aura quite oppressive.

There was no way to help this man with the medical condition he claimed disabled him. He did not want help. His problem was not medical; it involved a personal agenda to get a form filled out so he could keep up whatever he was doing while getting paid for that which he was not doing. I cannot emphasize enough that pain is invisible. Numbness and tingling and burning are invisible. It is exactly because of this subjective nature of these sensations that the interaction between patient and physician is critical. The doctor has to believe the patient is telling the truth, and the patient has to trust that the doctor is listening and believing. Barriers to this human interplay block the power of the goodwill possible between the two people. I truly wondered, if Jesus Christ had stood before this man on that day and offered to relieve whatever discomfort was paralyzing his hands, would the man have simply repeated that he needed his form filled out? Real people watched real miracles performed by

Jesus, watched real dead people be raised from the dead, and they still did not believe. It *is* possible to be so hard-hearted.

Encountering evil has a way of making you feel trapped, distracted, uncertain, and suspicious. These emotions don't work well in the intimacy of a therapeutic relationship, or in any relationship based on, and presuming, trust between the participants. I am not talking about mere awkwardness between people, or the realization that people aren't quite clicking, or simply don't like each other. I am referring to a manipulative aspect of one person toward another that seeks to damage or injure the other or put the other in a severely vulnerable position. So often the Pharisees' interactions with Christ are described in this way. They were continuously scheming to trick him in situations that on the surface appeared to be about healing the sick or discussing religious matters. Christ "knew what was in their hearts" each time. He would try to teach them and enlighten them, but he would most often be distressed or disappointed by their refusal to open their hearts and minds to the truths he offered.

Unfortunately, this dynamic is at work in some patients. No matter what explanations are given for their continued pain or what treatment options are offered to help, some patients establish an adversarial position with their doctors. The doctor is the enemy. The enemy is to be cornered, challenged, threatened, and doubted at all times.

Certain patients have hunkered down so far within themselves that their pain is no longer the issue. What is really at stake is their power. In their minds, control is paramount. Their pride in being correct about their conditions is more important than are any dealings with the conditions themselves. The thing I look for on the part of patients, even difficult ones, is a *genuine interest* in getting better, in getting on with their lives in some way. People in pain who convey no such interest cannot be helped except perhaps through prayer and psychology, the latter which they will rarely accept. However, doctors, nurses, and staff must be careful not to dismiss people because their imperfections just happen to be too distasteful.

The Value of Psychology

One of the hardest challenges I have as a physician is getting patients to consider psychological expertise and counseling as a component of their treatment. For the most part, we attribute to psychology a stigma of failure on our parts that is much more difficult to accept than any perceived physical failing. We look at recommendations for psychological consultations as direct evidence of our dysfunction as persons. A million things may be falling apart around us as we try to deal with serious illness or crushing pain, yet we never think or admit that maybe our minds and our psyches could use a little assistance.

Somehow we find it harder to believe that there is professional expertise out there that can offer insights for dealing with emotional/non-physical challenges than to believe that there is some surgery or medicine that will make the problems themselves go away. It is amazing how often and how many patients call in for more narcotic pain medicine when their lives become more stressful or filled with crises. To be sure, their pain tolerance may be down temporarily. But I tell them opiates are for the pain in their lives, not for their painful lives themselves.

Accepting help from a counselor, psychologist, or psychiatrist can be the strongest action you can take in facilitating health and healing in the face of pain and suffering. Accepting pain as sacrifice does not preclude asking a psychologist for advice on how to make it easier on your family. Depression as a result of chronic pain is not a defeat but a normal physiologic response to the unremitting assault of disease and the physicochemical process of pain. Allow yourself to accept that some things you never have believed in may actually be of value, may be worth looking at, may in fact work.

Likewise, allow yourself to accept that some things you have always believed in may not be the best for you right now, may not be effective in your current circumstances, may have given you all that they can give in your present situation. If you believe that God has created all that exists, then believe that God provides all sorts of tools for you to work with—you cannot possibly have known and tried all of them.

When Jesus walked on this earth, he probably didn't have a halo, some obvious sign that he was the person to follow. Many people missed the miracles because they were looking for someone who didn't look like Jesus. That someone for you may be a kind, discerning therapist, or a psychiatrist trained to help you manage the chemical chaos in your head that is the result of ongoing pain and fatigue.

The Other Side of Resistance

Finally, we have to acknowledge that evil sometimes resides in a caregiver: the doctor, nurse, therapist, clergy, or family member. They are the ones who may be acting out of the need to dominate or control others. Their technical brilliance may be wielded in ways that dehumanize patients or rob vulnerable people of their dignity. The power itself is not the evil. In fact, we approach the power of God or the power of an expert because we seek to access it. But just as doctors must be sensitive to the emotions elicited within them by certain patients, you must beware of the emotions generated within you by those to whom you are about to entrust your health, your body, and your life. You must be comfortable in being vulnerable to your caregivers. This allows healing to take place.

Some people are referred to doctors whose personalities don't match theirs or who simply don't have great bedside manners. Some patients value these things more than others. Many patients figure that if the doctor is good, or is the best expert specialist, or is trusted by the doctor who referred them in the first place, they'll tolerate the less-than-perfect human interaction in exchange for a successful outcome.

Being vulnerable in your need for care, you still must not be blind to caregivers who seek to take advantage of that vulnerability or who are dismissive of you as a person. You are always equal to others as a person, in any encounter, even when you are not an equal in knowledge or expertise. You must judge when a doctor is simply tired and in a bad mood, as opposed to when he or she is being truly cold and lacking in compassion. We hope that true evil is just as rare in caregivers as it is in patients, but remember the Pharisees and those others in the Gospels who could be so cruel to the vulnerable. Some doctors unfortunately fall short on personality, social skills, communication abilities, or simple likability. But if your gut tells you something is more seriously wrong, listen to it. If you feel too disconnected from the other person, find someone else. It is, after all, your health, your body, and your life.

Sometimes patients have been hurt too badly by life, by failure of medical care, or by the reactions they perceive in people around them. Their defense has been to grow resistant, self-centered, and heartless. They cannot overcome the anger and evil that has festered within them as a result. Evil can always be overcome by good, but not necessarily the good offered at a particular time or by a particular person. God is always open to us. The freedom granted to us by our Creator allows us to choose at any time to reopen a hardened heart or forgive a heart hardened against us.

I Pray Now for the Time When . . .

Lord, I fear I don't even recognize the evil I have within me.
Will I awaken one day, in some timeless space, to find myself alone,
    wondering where everyone and everything else has gone?
Will I be left with the person about whom I seemed to care most
    during my life—myself?

I pray you never let me drift from you.
I fear that somehow in my weakness or greed or bitterness,

I may somehow abandon you.
Save me from myself then, O Lord.

I know you have created goodness in me,
Do not allow the sufferings and weariness,
the disappointments and trials in this life,
to strip away that goodness,
and leave me distant from you.

If I am too lost to find my way back to you,
please send guides to show me the path.
Do not let them give up on me,
Even if I hurt them and lash out and rage at them in my
*   brokenness.*
Do not let them shake the dust of my life from their sandals and
*   leave me to myself.*

I pray now for the time when I may not have the heart left in me to
*   pray.*
Save me then, as I pray to be saved now.
And I ask the same for all those I love.
If I am to be your instrument for another,
let me not be frightened away
by the evil I fear may hurt me.
Let us each love one another, as you have loved us.
So that into your hands we may commend our spirits.

Questions for Your Health

- *Evil* is such a strong word. Can you recognize its hold on you in any way? How might it affect your recovery and healing?

- Have you ever felt totally cold toward your caregivers? The tough question is whether the impetus was within you and why.

• None of us is perfect, but if you feel that your long illness and suffering have begun to eat away at the goodness within you and lessen your sincere desire to stay connected to God, then you need to admit it, put aside your pride, and ask forgiveness. "I'm sorry" and "You're forgiven" are two of the most powerful healing statements on earth.

12

"AND JESUS WEPT."

The Journey through
Sorrow and Death

My God, my God, why have you forsaken me? . . . O my God, I cry by day, but you do not answer; and by night, but find no rest.

Psalm 22 (NRSV)

After Jesus asked where his deceased friend had been laid, the Gospel of John reports simply, "And Jesus wept." In Luke 19:41, Jesus' heart broke over Jerusalem and its people to whom he had given himself: "As he drew near, he saw the city and he wept over it." Perhaps he wept over all people, to whom he always gives himself.

We come to the story of death and dying. Loss of life does not necessarily mean only the physical death of a person. For many, the loss of a loved one, especially a spouse or child, is worse than the death of self. Even the loss of a loved one through a relationship that dies can seem more devastating than the death of self. Physical pain can be so torturous that some individuals would rather end their present lives than remain in its unbearable, unrelenting grasp.

Nevertheless, this life is all we know. We do not know, in spite of what we believe, what comes after this life. Letting go of self or of another into death is a wrenching process. If dying is so natural to life, why do we fight and fear it so?

Christians believe that we are born ultimately to return in death to our home in God. This seems to make the intervening life on earth even more the mystery and puzzle. Why are we here at all in this temporary existence, and why are we so attached to these bodies of ours and to our mundane routines? Wouldn't we want to be rid of all our suffering and limitations? Why then do death and dying seem to be such dreadful intrusions? Yet they are. We are perhaps always fending off death subconsciously.

Likewise, in the Gospels, death is associated with much sadness and lamenting. Jesus often seeks to reframe the event or to teach us the triumph of eternal life over earthly death. Throughout the Gospel stories, he tries to teach us that death is not something to be feared, even if sometimes it is portrayed as a day of reckoning. Yet he does not negate death's impact on those who suffer the loss of loved ones. He takes pity and has mercy. He takes pity on the mother in the burial procession of her son. He follows distraught parents and masters when they beg him to heal their children or their servants. And, again, we all know the story of his life-giving response to the death of his friend Lazarus, brother of Martha and Mary.

Surviving the Deaths of Those We Love

As a doctor, I have seen many people die right in front of me. I have also seen the birth of disabled babies. I have seen the loss of full and healthy lives by car accidents or diving accidents, young men and women left paralyzed or brain injured. Older individuals have become instantly helpless in the devastating flash of a stroke. I've known children who would remain forever childlike after a near-drowning incident. All these entail, in some manner, a loss of life. But death itself is a special grief and journey.

I have lost two of my closest friends to deaths in their young-adult years. They both fought the good fight. I was witness to each of them leaving this life to pass into the mystery of whatever is next.

Julie had dark, flashing eyes and a quick smile. She was pretty, yet so easygoing. She was a great friend to all of us and brought many people together. What a wonderful wife and mother she would have been. She ran a little bookstore until it closed, then went off to work at a law office before managing an architectural tour boat company.

Tour boats don't do well in the frozen waters around Chicago in the winter, so she escorted one of them down to a temporary port on Florida's Captiva Island. But she didn't stay long because she developed a cough, and they sent her home with a chest X-ray and a CAT scan.

I remember to this day the afternoon she handed those films to me in her living room and said, "Okay, Doctor Dan, what is it? Am I going to die? Is that a fur ball in my chest or is that cancer?"

I could feel my own face go ashen as I held the films up to her ceiling light. I was bewildered for a few seconds, as I could not even tell which way to turn them. You see, a chest X-ray is one of the more basic radiological films to orient because the large silhouette of the heart is always in the lower left lung field. The lung fields themselves should otherwise appear as dark domed rectangles. As I struggled with my puzzlement while trying to look like her expert doctor friend, I figured out the reason: she had a mass so large in her right lung that its white opacity mirrored the size and shape of her heart on the left side. It was growing out of or up into what is called the mediastinum, the area between the lungs, under the sternum. Though I tried to hide my face behind the films I was holding up, I knew she could already see the wobble in my stance, perhaps the very wobble in me, as I was hit with the shock wave: I was going to lose my dear Julie.

Well, she had her treatments, her bout with steroid psychosis, her puffiness, her hair loss and wigs. She battled through with strength and humor, writing to me in Boston (where I was in a six-month fellowship) when she had the energy, searching for God's voice through the storm's howling wind. Then it became calm. Her doctor announced that she had reached remission. She didn't need a checkup for three to six months. For her, it was like waking from the bad dream, those first few weeks of balmy, breezy, blue-sky June days. As we know even after being laid up with a cold or the flu, it's amazing how the simplest pleasures are retasted with utmost heightened sensitivity. Every sight and touch is precious, and relished.

It was not to last. She fell ill again that summer within a couple of months, and tests showed recurrences. New doctors and new treatments were pulled out of the oncology arsenal. Her system was shelled and blasted with all the salvos the medical guns could bring to bear. But the guns weren't all that accurate back then, and despite good intent, her liver and kidneys took some friendly fire. She twice needed painful chest-tube placements to drain fluid from around her lungs to help her breathe.

She had a brief respite from her battling in November of 1987, but I believe she knew the enemy was staging its final assault and that the fall could be imminent. Though she didn't outwardly concede, she took this time to give each of us some crystallized insights on life and, in particular, on our own lives as they had blended with hers.

She did not mince words. She did not have the time to be flowery and indirect. She was letting us in on her view from the edge— the very edge—of the life she had left to share. Who knows how life looks until one is granted the awareness of its impending end and can see that a transition is coming on fast.

The last time I heard her voice was on the phone; she was back in the hospital, short of breath, angry in a smart-aleck way at God for not letting up on her. She was told she needed another chest tube, which she hated, and was scheduled for it that afternoon. I wanted to see her because I was leaving for a week away with my father. I feared going away. She insisted she would be fine and absolutely forbade me from coming in and seeing her in her unkempt and haggard state. "I'll see you when you get back and I'm out of this damn hospital." Good-bye.

When I returned home a week later, I had a message on my answering machine calmly telling me to call the hospital when I got in that day. It was 10:30 p.m. on a Friday. Julie's best girlfriend Terry answered the phone in the hospital hall and hit me with, "She must be waiting for you. The rest of us are all here. Paul just got in today. You're the only one who needs to get here. She's been in a coma since Tuesday. Joan (her mom) won't let them turn off the ventilator till everyone is here, and Doctor Dan, you're the only one not here yet."

After driving to the hospital in a state of blankness I had never experienced, I found her room. The circle of friends and family was waiting around her bed, with a space open for me. I felt like the key that locked the chain of finality around her leaving. We were there to hold her and to hold one another. Her mother looked up from her place by Julie's head, holding her hand, and smiled at me bravely, inviting me to come over and say good-bye to her beautiful Julie.

Another friend, Father Terry, said a prayer. We all bade her farewell. She would not be coming back home this night but would leave by another route. So the ventilator was turned off, and we watched the green line on the monitor pulse down to a few final gentle undulations. The ripples disappeared then as into the flat surface of a small green pond. "Look," said one in the circle of crying loved ones, "she's smiling." And sure enough, her face had relaxed into that angelic look of peace and relief and permission: all was okay. It said to us, "You have all been wonderful friends and family. You are free to live. I am fine." It was around two or three in the morning. It was the Feast of Our Lady of Guadalupe, December 12, 1987.

Fighting Till the End

I met Patrick in the seventh grade when I moved to a new school. We became best friends. His mother became my mother, and my mother became his. We transitioned from giggling boys goofing off to maddening teenagers waiting on each other's porches till the day we could drive, through the challenges of all those teenage years, on into adulthood. I was best man at his wedding and confirmation sponsor for his eldest son. I didn't expect to share with him so soon the moments leading up to his death.

Patrick was never one for expressing his feelings, and that trait turned into a real stoicism as he grew into manhood and became a husband and father. He always had fun, but he took on a bit of the John Wayne persona, strong and silent. This characterized a fight he would wage against cancer for eleven years. He was diagnosed with a melanoma when he was in his mid-twenties. Melanoma, being the most serious form of skin cancer, was treated aggressively with surgery and whatever form of supplemental treatments was required to eradicate any suspected spread.

Patrick actually did quite well and made it past the magic five-year survival mark. But unfortunately, so had some of the cancer cells, and they reappeared two years after the all-clear signal. They showed up in the form of lymph nodes swollen in his groin. He went through another surgery and aggressive treatments. His leg would now be prone to swelling because the surgery altered the circulation drainage. But he was doing okay again, stoically following all the doctor's orders. No real big discussions on feelings or fears. He kept up his job and his community commitments, continued helping his wife raise their three children and take care of their home. As much as possible, they kept his cancer a tiny blip on the radar screen.

But within a few more years, eleven since the original diagnosis, the final battle began, and this one was not to be won. The cancer had taken up key positions all around his body, and the treatments available could not overcome it. Patrick strode on through life. He went with his wife to Lourdes as part of a "do it now" trip around Europe. Otherwise, he kept working and being active as long as he could.

When he began to weaken physically, he decided he would spend as much time at home as possible, and little or no time in any hospital. When I spoke with him a few weeks before he died, he stayed superficial and light about his situation, preferring to ask about me or to talk about sports. But Patrick had always been like that. I hadn't expected otherwise but wanted to give him room to talk if he wished. I don't think he was conceding yet, but adapting to the limits being forced upon him. Onward Christian soldier, marching as to war . . .

Holy Week and Good Friday of 1995 coincided with the cancer's overwhelming final assault, and I was back in Cincinnati from Chicago to be there. The pain required morphine, which made him drowsy and punchy. The cancer had spread to the lungs, liver, bone, and brain. Hospice was helping. There were no plans to enter the hospital. He was fighting this one out on his home field. Friends and family took turns at the bedside. Nerves were frayed as fears of the end collided with prayers for his relief.

He was able to receive communion on Easter Sunday, eyes closed, dutifully folding his hands as he had when he and I were altar boys together. In twenty-four hours, he would be meeting face-to-face the God he now took in the tiny Host from the priest. So amazing to contemplate such a part of our faith: do we believe it? I think Patrick did, in his very black-and-white, no-questions-asked, follow-orders kind of way. He just wasn't ready to go yet. He had a family he did not want to leave. But God was insistent.

Somehow Patrick clawed his way through those last twelve hours. I could see his stubbornness, even in the context of his respect for the God who was waiting for him. God let him take whatever time he needed. After all, it had been eleven years. There was no rush, except for those of us watching the tremendous struggle, especially his mortally wounded mother, who could not concede to God either. She had no power but to watch her son suffer, all the more because of his strong will to not succumb.

His fighting brought him all the more pain, yet he battled on. He would not give in to make it easier on himself. He would not concede if he could hang on for the miracle. He would have to be taken, because he was not leaving voluntarily. He, I think, felt it was his noble and sacrificial duty to remain at his guard-post for his family no matter what. It was stubbornness of personality turned to valor of heroism. It was life doing to the utmost what it was created to do—live to the brink of all it was allotted, and not one second, literally not one, sooner. And it would cease only because its creator, its source of breath, would come to carry it off—to somewhere distant and unknown to the eyes of those left behind, yet somewhere beautiful and safe in the faith of our eternal souls.

I have witnessed many things in my life, but none as incredible as those final few minutes. Had I seen an ascension? Truly, it was as if the ceiling opened above that bed and all the power of heaven came down to rescue Patrick from his own will to remain in his suffering rather than surrender to the love of God. I have heard others tell me of their similar experiences with family members. In a way, this life possesses us. It takes an exorcism of sorts to free us from its hold.

Though our religious faith tells us we should not be so tied to this earthly life, we cling to it instinctively. This is natural. It is not an evil we hold onto. It is the gift of God, which we then must somehow allow ourselves to hand back over to him, in trust that we are being led to something more complete, rich, and fulfilling.

A loved one's death takes a lot out of those keeping vigil. The ones at the bedside will not have the feel of God's saving arms around them at the dying moment. We believe the deceased to be swept up into the glorious ecstasy of God's love. Those of us who remain are left in a chasm of pain and loss, and in a challenge called faith. Darkness and coldness can block any previous trust in the warmth of God's love and mercy. God has taken this life from us, and we have no heart left with which to plead any help from that distant, unhearing power. We are broken, because no deliverance came, and there was no miracle.

Six Who Faced Death, Knowing Jesus

In the Gospels, there are six people who, one could say, faced their own deaths as they interacted with Jesus. First was Simeon, who, after waiting his entire life to see the presence of God, finally recognized it in the baby Jesus brought to the temple by Mary and Joseph. Then there was John the Baptist, awaiting an uncertain fate in prison, before he was beheaded. The two thieves crucified on either side of Jesus present two powerfully different approaches to death. And then Peter and John discuss their fates with the risen Christ.

Simeon

Simeon was a man who looked forward in hope. "This man was righteous and devout, awaiting the consolation of Israel, and the holy Spirit was upon him. It had been revealed to him by the holy Spirit that he should not see death before he had seen the Messiah of the Lord" (Luke 2:25–26). Here was a man whose life of prayer and faithfulness had led him to be so certain of the existence of his God that he was promised a vision of the Son of God before he died. In some ways, this also meant that he would be notified of his death.

Who of us truly wants to know the date and time of our death? Though the uncertainty of death is a huge part of what leads us to fear it, are we faith-filled enough to handle the knowledge of its imminence? When facing a grave illness, we want some sense from our doctors of what to expect. Whether for practical planning, for psychological acceptance, or for spiritual preparation, gaining some sense of what we are up against and how much more time we can reasonably expect to live is, for most people, very helpful. It allows us some control over a process about which we otherwise don't have too much say. Yet it is an awesome knowledge to bear.

John the Baptist

After being thrown into prison, John the Baptist, Jesus' own cousin, who spent his entire life preaching of the coming of the Messiah, faced the uncertainty of his own future and perhaps expected he would be executed:

When John heard in prison of the works of the Messiah, he sent his disciples to him with this question, "Are you the one who is to come, or should we look for another?" (Matthew 11:2–3)

John is expressing a genuine desire to be sure of Christ. His search is true and sincere, and that is the message for us, even to the moment of our deaths. But he still seeks assurance. He perhaps wants to know that his life has not been lived in vain. This question is the last line spoken by John in the Gospels. Christ sends him back an answer of hope, that the lame are walking, the blind are seeing, the poor are receiving the Good News. "John, it is okay. You have done well. You have chosen the right path. All is as it should be." The next time we hear of John the Baptist he has been beheaded.

When they are faced with the diagnosis of terminal cancer with only so many months to live, many people become very direct and intimate with God regarding questions about life and faith. Expressing our doubts genuinely allows God to enlighten us. In this way, our remaining time can be spent in anticipation of going to God in honesty, openness, and reconciliation. This sort of encounter makes it more possible for fear to be lessened, guilt relieved, and anger shed. After we have dealt honestly with God, we can look forward in hope, as did John the Baptist.

The Two Thieves

Luke's Gospel provides the most detail about the two thieves crucified with Christ. One of the dying men, perhaps in his desperation, panic, and torment on the cross, demands that Jesus use his messianic powers to save them. Luke says that he "blasphemed" in this demand, indicating a less-than-sympathetic interpretation of the man's motives. We can sense that this man did not truly care about Jesus and that the potential power to save them all from their predicaments did not interest him in any way other than self-preservation.

The other thief—who has since been named St. Dismas—was incredulous at the attitude taken by the first thief, even at the brink of death and judgment. "Have you no fear of God, for you are subject to the same condemnation?" (Luke 23:40). This man, under the exact same stresses of pain and suffering, facing the same existential annihilation, chose to acknowledge his own sinfulness and throw his future onto the mercy of the man Jesus, whom he perceived to be powerful and good. "We have been condemned justly, for the sentence we received corresponds to our crimes, but this man has done nothing criminal." Then he said, "Jesus, remember me when you come into your kingdom" (Luke 23:41–42).

As we face the inevitability of death, or the unrelenting pain of a long dying process, in spite of our fears and our desires to be saved, do we choose to accept our condition? Do we give our lives and sufferings over to the mercy and care of God, or do we thrash about demanding to be saved, to be spared what all others, and even God himself, are destined to go through? As with all the issues spoken of in this book, I am making a critical distinction here between the fears and emotional reactions natural to stressful suffering and an essential hardness of heart.

In this hanging between life and the unknown hereafter, one man turned to love, in remorse for whatever he might have done wrong in life, and hoped in something greater to come. He didn't quite know what that meant; he just asked to be remembered when Jesus came into his reign. Unlike some of the apostles, he did not ask for a high seat at Jesus' right or left hand. He simply placed his trust in Jesus' mercy.

This might have been one of the most, if not the most, intimate moments of Jesus' human life. In the aloneness that each of us will experience at the approach of death, the words of others standing at the same doorstep may be more assuring than anyone else's, even those of people most dear to us. This thief, like the leper early in the Gospels, in the midst of all the suffering and agony, recognized Jesus in some profound way for who he really was. This led Jesus to turn to him and to respond as the source of love, mercy, and triumph over death.

Jesus did not upset the natural order of things by what he said. These three men were going to die their physically horrible deaths. But Jesus assures us in the words he gives to this dying thief that he is truly merciful, even though he rescued none of them from their present moments of pain. In doing so, he shows us that life is more than what we are able to see of it.

One of the most precious, saving, hope-engendering lines of the entire Bible is the reply Jesus gave to this man: "I say to you: today you will be with me in Paradise" (Luke 23:43). *This is our God* speaking to each of us, from the cross, from the center of the universe, from the focal point, the very end for which he was born! He says, "It's not over! I have won. I have won all for you. Death is not the end. You will not be annihilated. Your loved ones are safe. Though you cannot yet see, I am telling you now, I am assuring you now, at this most damned moment in all history, that love triumphs. Life lives on. YOU will live on. Today! This VERY DAY. In paradise."

Can we believe in those words at every death of a loved one, at every tragic event we see or hear about in our greater connection with humanity? Jesus assures us that a greater life awaits us. There is no game playing with this "good thief" as both he and Jesus hang on their crosses, suffocating, agonizing, dying. Jesus says definitively, to the thief and to each of us, "You will be with me this day in paradise."

May we truly take these words of solace to heart at every deathbed, every wake, every funeral, every graveside. If we did, somehow I think we wouldn't suffer so much in the rest of our lives. Do you think these words of Christ changed everything about the final hours of this man's pain on the cross? Did they make breathing easier? Did they make the man's legs any stronger or his feet hurt any less as he was forced to press down on them to get a breath? Did they dull the burning nerve pain in his arms and the aching in his shoulders as he struggled to raise his body to catch another breath? Did they even calm his fears of how much worse the pain could get or the uncertainty of what dying would feel like?

He and Christ likely still suffered the human physical aspects of their dying. What I believe God's promise did do for this man, and what it can do for us, was to tell him his pain and suffering would end, offering as much absoluteness to the fulfillment of his hopes as was possible in such a moment. Pain is terrible often because of its uncertain duration and intensity and because of our inability to control it.

The "bad" thief and the "good" thief likely suffered the same physical pains and the same physiological processes as they died. The "good" thief, however, had the hope of a victory in spite of his physical defeat and imminent annihilation. He was not *spiritually* defeated. He had the gift of hope that he would not be vanquished by what he was going through. His counterpart, however, could not see beyond himself, nor beyond the immediacy of his own suffering. He was left to go through the dying alone in his own anguished, angry, bitter mind.

Peter

When Jesus appears to his apostles after the Resurrection, he says to Peter:

> *"Amen, amen, I say to you, when you were younger, you used to dress yourself and go where you wanted; but when you grow old, you will stretch out your hands, and someone else will dress you and lead you where you do not want to go."* He said this signifying by what kind of death he would glorify God. (John 21:18–19)

Peter's only response is to turn around and notice that John is there also. He asks Jesus the very natural and blunt question, "Lord, what about him?" (John 21:21). Jesus challenges him with the hypothetical question, "What if I want him to remain until I come? What concern is it of yours? You follow me" (John 21:22). (Tradition has it that John was the only apostle to die a natural death rather than die through martyrdom.)

We come back again to the question of whether you would live your life differently if you knew when and how you were going to die. Jesus says to us what he said to Peter: "What difference would it make? Your business is to follow me." Can we answer Jesus that we are living our lives right now the way we would if our doctors told us today we had six months to live?

If we are living essentially different lives from the ones we would live if suddenly given the news of a terminal illness, then Jesus might want us to step aside with him to have a talk, as he did with Peter. "Do you love me? Then live out that love in your life, starting now."

We could perhaps fear death less if it were to come for each of us as a distant quiet sleep, long from now when we are old and ready to fade tired into the night. If it was guaranteed to arrive gently, without pain or trauma, and we had accomplished all we had wanted to in life, we might be able to face it at least a little better. Yet death too often intrudes while we are busy going about our living and our loving. It can come with terror, violence, and pain. It snatches us or our loved ones long before we are ready to say good-bye.

The more we fear death, though, the more we seek to avoid it, and such efforts will determine everything else about life. It could lead to cautious behavior, preventing us from acting on insights and wisdom that might put our lifestyle at risk. Or, in the opposite way, it could lead us to live gluttonously, trying to defeat death by hoarding more of life. But our lives should have the same integrity, motivation, and direction, whatever the calendar allots us.

Lazarus

Finally, let us notice again the tenderness of Jesus in the face of others' death and dying. The most well-known story about death in the Gospels, other than Christ's own, is the raising of Lazarus in the Gospel of John. Jesus was aware of what he was about to do for

Lazarus. But does Jesus' knowledge and intent make it any easier on Lazarus as he experiences dying, or on his sisters and other friends as they watch helplessly, wondering where Jesus the healer, Jesus their friend, is?

Where is our God, they lament in tears and prayer, as Lazarus slips away. The mothers of my dying friends Julie and Patrick likely wailed the same cries in their hearts. How can he stay away when the one he loves, the one I love, is dying? Does God show up because we have pushed the "call button" at the bedside? No, he is already with us and does not have to come running from anywhere in order to reach us.

Rather, it is we who have to discern God's presence in the various events of our lives. The fear of death will suddenly put the fear of God in us. The moment we find out we have cancer or a loved one is dying in an emergency room of a heart attack or of injuries from an auto accident, we forget about whatever had us distracted throughout our lives up to now and focus quite suddenly on "Where is God? Someone find him. Hurry—I need him now!"

Martha and Mary, who knew Jesus in the flesh, acknowledged him as the Messiah, and professed belief in the resurrection of the dead on the last day, still cried to Jesus that they missed their brother. They presumed he would not have died if Jesus had been there. Yet God *was* as present to Martha and Mary at the time of Lazarus's dying as he *is to us* every moment of our lives, even when we beg him to come quickly. Though we say the same words of faith, we, too, still wish for Jesus to save our loved ones from dying.

You probably have not talked much about death with your doctor or members of your family. At least allow yourself to pray to God about it. Risk the inner shudder it may produce, but trust that our Lord will be gentle with you. When it is your time, he may still have to wrench you unto himself, as with my friend Patrick, or you may gently slip out from the circle of your friends and family, as did my friend Julie. Remember Simeon, John the Baptist, the good thief, Peter, and Lazarus. Read their stories again to discern God's message to you about the mystery of your own life and whatever fears you may have about this transition we call death.

Jesus himself promises us paradise at the end of our pain, as he did directly with the good thief. He gives meaning to the sacrifices we make throughout life in choosing to follow him, as he assured his cousin John. He shows us through Simeon how to gently, fearlessly welcome both life and death through the revelations of God. He challenges us, as he did Peter, to live fully, even in the awareness of an end to life. Do not live out of fear, intimidation, or distractions. Jesus says to us, live your life the same, whether it be long or short.

Jesus' *entire* documented life was lived with the awareness that he was going to die. "It is for this that I have come into the world." He experienced his own agony in the Garden of Gethsemane, where he openly expressed his anguish before the final moments. For the love of every single human being, each one a creation of His, in a divine miracle He would take on the suffering of all and share in it.

Let us look closely at how Jesus lived. He enjoyed being with people. He taught people how to live in peace with one another. He encouraged each person to live the fullest life possible. He did not worry about making money. He did not engage in political revolution, though he did always seek to stir up a revolution of the heart and soul. He did not act out of self-protection, but instead spoke boldly of justice and compassion and of God, even from the time he was twelve. Awareness of death did not lead him to avoid or to hoard. He walked with an "abandonment of the heart" toward others and toward God, in an image, relayed to me by a friend, from Charles de Foucauld. Even when his disciples were dismayed that he would risk going to Jerusalem, knowing the danger that awaited him there, Jesus walked into the next moment of life as he had all others—fully, without holding back any part of himself. Eternity is now. There is no waiting. Life is here where you are, even if "here" is your moment of dying. Do you love me? Feed my lambs.

Show me, Lord, that you are here.
For the very gift you give me to think freely
Causes me to consider that I may in fact be alone.

It is written in Isaiah,
That you have my name carved in the palm of your hand.
I pray to always trust in your care for me, freeing me to care for
    others.

I believe you yourself hung on the cross as man
Searching the forlorn gray skies for yourself as God
Perhaps knowing the doubts I feel as a weak, fearful creature.

You are the very love that holds the world.
You are the very certainty into which you gave yourself from the
    cross.
Into your hands may I learn to commend my own spirit, each day,
    and on my last day.

It is I who as yet look through a glass darkly.
May I see the Kingdom you reminded John to see.
It is all around me, even now.

I pray, therefore, Lord, to run full speed through life, not fearing
    death,
And to splash through the end into your arms,
As through a mere cascade of cleansing water.

May we each burst into the glorious sunshine of your heaven.
You yourself told us it was Paradise.
How then can it not be so?

Amen

Questions for Your Health

- It is a bit scary to hear Christ's words that unless we die like a grain of wheat we cannot grow. Have you ever said out loud, "I am afraid of dying," if in fact you are? To a priest or minister, to a doctor, to a spouse or friend? To yourself? What image do you have of death—something that threatens, or relieves, or something else?

- Whatever the image of death you carry, does it give you peace and enable you to live more fully, or does it leave you anxious and cause you to live restlessly? How do we die to ourselves a little each day, and thus learn to live more freely the lives we have?

- Imagine being told you will die two weeks from today, or one year from today. Name two things you would do differently starting now. Name three things you would keep doing the same. Can you name why you are not doing the first two?

- If you are young, imagine yourself elderly. If you are old, imagine yourself in your youth. Have a gentle conversation with yourself—are you happy with who you were or who you see yourself becoming? Can the older say to the younger, don't worry, you're doing all right, it will all work out, you are on the right path? Can the younger say to the older, I am proud of what you did with the gift of your life. I understand and appreciate the efforts and sacrifices you have made. I will live my life to become like you.

- Finally do you even sense a "heaven"? Do you believe God loves you enough to bring you home to him, no matter your strivings or your imperfections? Do you trust that all your loved ones are safe in their destinies, and can you, in that faith, leave them in God's eternal care, even though you would, or already do, miss them terribly? Would you live differently or suffer differently now if you truly believed this? If not, what is leading you to doubt? If it is your own sinfulness, do you doubt, like Judas, that Jesus is strong enough to redeem even the likes of you? If it is just doubt in what you cannot see, can you dare trying to see that which you would most deeply desire?

13

"A SWORD OF SORROW SHALL PIERCE YOUR HEART."

The Mystery Called Suffering

It is not as though there are two paths, one the way of the cross and the other the way of resurrection victory. Rather, the resurrection means that the way of the cross is the way of victory.

Jesus did not suffer and die in order that we need not suffer and die, but in order that our suffering and death might be joined to his in redemptive victory.

The Christian way is not one of avoidance but of participation in the suffering of Christ, which encompasses not only our own suffering, but the suffering of the whole world.

Richard John Neuhaus, *Death on a Friday Afternoon*

The ultimate question we ask is, Why do we have to suffer at all? Why is there pain in the first place? Why do we have to die? The majority of us, even in our efforts to be people of faith, still experience hurts to our bodies, anguish in our emotions, and grieving of great losses here on earth, not in some timeless eternity. We still see wars, natural disasters, and accidents as wastes, as events that should not have happened. We lament those who die too young. We are pierced by the sword of sorrow, and cannot remove it.

First, the Questions Restated

Rabbi Harold S. Kushner wrote *When Bad Things Happen to Good People* after watching his child go through the slow process of dying. He tried to reconcile his view of God's involvement in our lives in the light of that difficult experience. His conclusion was that God does not cause suffering. Suffering is the consequence of the free universe. Suffering is impersonal and amoral in how it is dispersed through the world, through history, and through each of our lives. God does not choose to inflict pain on one person over the other:

> Can you accept the idea that some things happen for no rea-son, that there is randomness in the universe? . . .
>
> Some people will find the hand of God behind everything that happens. . . .
>
> "In the beginning," the Bible tells us, "God created the heaven and the earth. The earth was formless and chaotic, with darkness covering everything." Then God began to work his creative magic on the chaos, sorting things out, imposing order where there had been randomness before. . . .
>
> But suppose God didn't quite finish by closing time on the afternoon of the sixth day? . . . Its six-day time frame is not meant to be taken literally. Suppose that Creation, the pro-cess of replacing chaos with order, were still going on. . . .
>
> It may yet come to pass that, as "Friday afternoon" of the world's evolution ticks toward the Great Sabbath which is the End of Days, the impact of random evil will be diminished.
>
> Or it may be that God finished his work of creating eons ago, and left the rest to us . . . In that case, we will simply have to learn to live with it, sustained and comforted by the knowledge that the earthquake and the accident, like the murder and the robbery, are not the will of God, but rep-resent that aspect of reality which stands independent of his

will, and which angers and saddens God even as it angers and saddens us.

In becoming human, he writes, we "entered the world of the knowledge of good and evil, a more painful, more complicated world," one in which we are self-conscious and will spend our lives making difficult choices. Our self-consciousness allows us to reflect on our experiences, our pasts, our hopes, and our pain, and thus leaves us vulnerable to suffering. Our free choosing allows us to hurt ourselves and others, through wrong choices or choices that conflict with others' or with the mere randomness of nature's events. Bad things then happen to good people.

Rabbi Kushner concludes that somehow God is powerless to stop the randomness of free will, and that he is angered and saddened by it, just as we are. On the last page of his book, he asks if we are "capable of forgiving and loving God" even when we have found out "that He is not perfect": "Even when He has let you down and disappointed you by permitting bad luck and sickness and cruelty in His world, and permitting some of those things to happen to you? Can you learn to love and forgive Him despite His limitations . . . ?"

Kushner suggests that we can view God as we do our parents, as someone from whom we have expected too much, someone we had always imagined as perfect and all powerful but who really is not. I choose to hope in God a different way. God is a mystery whose love I cannot yet explain. As one who sees God in Christ, I strive to discern his all-powerful goodness, undefeated even in suffering and death.

Another writer, Nicholas Wolterstorff, also tries to break out of the isolation of grief and suffering caused by his son's death, by sharing his pain in *Lament for a Son*. Wondering on God's role, he writes:

> I cannot fit it all together by saying, "He [God] did it," but neither can I do so by saying, "There was nothing he could do about it." I cannot fit it together at all. I can only, with

Job, endure. I do not know why God did not prevent Eric's death. To live without the answer is precarious. It's hard to keep one's footing.

Eric is gone, here and now he is gone; now I cannot talk with him, now I cannot see him, now I cannot hug him, now I cannot hear of his plans for the future. That is my sorrow. A friend said, "Remember, he's in good hands." I was deeply moved. But that reality does not put Eric back in my hands now. That's my grief. For that grief, what consolation can there be other than having him back?

Suffering is down at the center of things, deep down where the meaning is. Suffering is the meaning of our world. For Love is the meaning. And Love suffers. The tears of God are the meaning of history. But mystery remains. Why isn't Love-without-suffering the meaning of things? Why is suffering-Love the meaning? Why does God endure his suffering? Why does he not at once relieve his agony by relieving ours?

Why is there a cross and passion, a Holy Thursday and a Good Friday? Why is it "good"? Why the sorrow and suffering at all? Why is there this "suffering-love"? Does Jesus save us from pain? Or does he save us *in* pain, and in triumph *beyond* our pain and his? In the book *God & Human Suffering,* author Douglas Hall writes that the promised Messiah surprises humanity by manifesting himself as one whose power "expresses itself unexpectedly in the weakness of love."

Jesus and Mary Suffer with Us

When we ask how God can allow pain and suffering, we need to first acknowledge that the Creator of all things is present everywhere and always. Thus pain and suffering cannot be separate from God. If we believe that God is life-imbuing Spirit, we do not view God as sitting on some distant throne. These images may have seeped into our minds thanks to the efforts of devoted artists portraying the Almighty King of the universe, the Ultimate Ruling Father, the New Zeus. God is not coldly watching our pain and suffering, detached and demanding. He is bigger than this life we know, and thus the world is *a part of* him, not *apart from* him.

A basic tenet of Christian faith is that the God of the universe came to this planet and lived as one of us. Notice that God chose to enter his creation just as it was. Jesus was born into hardship. God's most perfect creation, the mother of Jesus, was caught up in a difficult situation regarding her pregnancy. The common people of the day turned away from their shelters a young mother in labor. A jealous king slaughtered babies in an attempt to kill this one future king he feared.

With the arrival of God into the very history of humanity, good and evil manifested themselves around him as they do around every other person in the world. God did not kill the children of Bethlehem. Herod and his soldiers did. Free human will, ego, and fear killed them.

Throughout the Gospels, Jesus acknowledged in so many ways the existence of both good and evil. He told stories that involved masters, slaves, and servants. He used images of kings and property owners, rich and poor, generals and armies, judges and prisons. He did not get rid of illness or death, even though he cured specific illnesses in specific people, and raised some from the dead. He did not get rid of the Romans or their dominance over Israel. Wars and catastrophes, crime and injustice happen. Our Lord did not eliminate injustice or cruelty or death as entities unto themselves. He preached against the evil in men's hearts that lead to these things.

The Scriptures indicated that his name was to be Emmanuel, "God *with* us," not "God *instead of* us." This is not an easy concept to grasp. Even Mary, believed by Catholics to be born sinless via the immaculate conception, struggled to understand the message of God, from the very first call to be God's portal into humanity.

When Jesus was born to her, she was foretold of a sword of sorrow that would pierce her heart, and that her son's life would be opposed by some in the world.

> Simeon blessed them and said to Mary his mother, ". . . (and you yourself a sword will pierce) so that the thoughts of many hearts may be revealed." (Luke 2:34–35)

Just a few passages later in Luke, twelve-year-old Jesus is found in the temple after Mary and Joseph have searched for him for three days. Mary asks, "Son, why have you done this to us? Your father and I have been looking for you with great anxiety" (Luke 2:48). Here is Mary questioning her son and her God as to why he was causing her to suffer! As a worried mother and perhaps as a symbol of all humanity, she sought in sorrow for her lost son, her lost God.

What of our own laments to God? When we pray and search for him with all our hearts, feeling helpless, can we look back on the heartbreaking search of Christ's own earthly mother? If she was told she would suffer a sword of sorrow and was confused in her own direct searching for her son who was God, how can we expect to escape suffering? And do we trust that he is fulfilling the "business" of being God for us, even though we cannot see him doing so?

"You Give Them Something to Eat"

Obviously, God could have merely appeared on earth; he did not need to be born. But he chose to enter the world through human birth. Creation was beautiful just as it was. God did not need to bypass it or avoid its "messy" parts. *This* is the life he created. *This* is the world over which he breathed his spirit. We are the people created in God's own likeness and image. The message seems to be that he did not come to change life itself but rather how we *live* it.

In the midst of free will and uncontrollable circumstances, how will you live the gift of the life given you? How will you handle the challenges you face or the opportunities you encounter? No matter how much we hear the words of Jesus, we still face everyday life and its irritations and unanswered questions. Just like the apostles, we have to be taught repeatedly to let go of our concerns for safety and comfort. Like them, we have to overcome our fear of pain. God doesn't remove our suffering but sometimes keeps us in the middle of it; in this way we learn how to live through it and help others do the same.

One day, when Jesus is surrounded by thousands and it is getting late, the apostles ask him to "dismiss the crowd" (Luke 9:12). How often would we rather have the needy sent away from us? We're uncomfortable with not only our own pain and poverty but that of others as well. How can we go about our busy lives—our vacations, home purchases, football games, or fancy dinners—when needy people are too close by?

Jesus answers them, "Give them some food yourselves" (Luke 9:13). The apostles are quick to defend themselves: "We have nothing but . . ." or "We only have these. . . ." or "How can we feed all these people?"

How does Jesus respond to their veiled excuses, or even just their simple fears? "You give them something to eat" (Mark 6:37 NRSV). You! "How many loaves do you have?" (Mark 6:38). Me? Well, but these are for me, I mean, well, it's for us. This isn't enough for all of them, too. What will we have left over for us? What will there be for me?

Jesus does not look at the scarcity, but the abundance. He looks outward, not inward. He gives thanks to his heavenly father. He does not give orders for the people, or the problem, to go away. Rather, he challenges his disciples to action, just as he challenges us. What will we do in the face of problems? He models for his disciples, for the crowds, and for us how to live through the problems.

After prodding his disciples to present what they themselves have, he gives the few loaves and fishes "to the disciples, who in turn

[give] them to the crowds" (Matthew 15:36). He allows his disciples to participate in the miracle of the sharing, the letting go, and the multiplying. He shows them how to give of what they have and thence to discover the abundance that God has already placed with them. He gives them the experience of making themselves part of the miracle. They learn that they are capable of using the power within themselves to bring good out of bad.

Jesus and his apostles did not get rid of hunger in the world or of hunger in the human condition. They did, however, alleviate hunger and suffering in that moment, for those people, in that place. Jesus did not react to the hunger around him by changing the hypothalamus region of the human brain in order to eliminate the biological drives called thirst and appetite. Nor does he eliminate wind and rain or the wonder of cellular reproduction, so that storms, floods, cancer, and infections can be avoided.

We hold onto a sense that there shouldn't be storms, floods, cancer, and infections. We accept free will, but we find it hard to accept its negative results. Was there an Eden without all this? Perhaps we carry within us a need for it to be so, or a memory of an eternal home from which we came, or that we remember, paradoxically, from our futures. Eternity is timelessness. It is always now. Perhaps we are in a perpetual state of déjà vu. Are we inspired by what we sense can be, or are we burdened and angered that life is not what we want, perfect, here and now?

The Voyage of Life

In the National Gallery in Washington, D.C., there hangs a four-painting series by Thomas Cole titled *The Voyage of Life*. Depicted in the first scene, subtitled "Childhood," is an idyllic, Edenic garden, through which flows a glassy, smooth stream, with blossoms cascading over the banks and floating on the water's surface. Out of the hollows of a dark cave to the left drifts a golden boat made of angels, upon which is nestled a gleeful baby, standing with arms outstretched, under the gaze of an angel whose hand easily guides the tiller of the boat. Rocky crags high above the cave drop off into a wide, sunny meadow. The boat glides into a world of lushness and color—the perfect picture of safety and divine nurturing love.

In the next frame is the depiction of the wondrous, limitless optimism of "Youth." Huge vistas of landscape and sky reach to the horizon. A lazy, winding path is taken by the flow of the stream, for of course there is all the time in the world to get where one wishes to go. The grassy banks are smooth, low, level, and accessible. Strong shade trees beckon for a springtime nap. The angel boat is dutifully helmed by the robust, ruddy, confident youth, as the angel guide who had steered for the babe now stands watchfully on the banks, allowing the youth his taste of control and independence.

Far ahead, a soft dirt road rises through the trees and hills in a distant land. High in the sky is an ethereal vision of a pearlescent palace, a symbol of grandiose dreams and larger-than-life achievement. Nearly hypnotized by the immensity of it all, Youth does not notice nor fear the hint of rougher waters at the distant course of the stream. He does not see that the waters beneath bend sharply away from the direction of his gaze. As yet, he does not hear or feel the rumbling of the rapids to come.

How suddenly the third scene of "Manhood" falls upon him, in a roaring deluge of rapids. The scene has transformed into a storm. The sky is churning and boiling with gray and black thunderheads. They personally blow their wrath upon his now tiny, frail craft, as the waters rush through a gauntlet of ragged rock. There are no flowers or lush gardens now. The only tree in the scene is twisted and split from the incessant tumult. There is no guiding vision in the sky. The angels that make up his boat are now themselves cowering at the impending plunge into waves down a rock-laden gorge.

Man stands before what seems to be the hostility of the entire world, hands supplicant in prayer, begging for mercy, yet looking up to a merciless, hidden heaven as the green waters rush into the foaming anger before him. What could await but certain death and destruction? He and his boat will be dashed to pieces. His guardian angel now hovers far above and behind him, a chasm seemingly light years away, observing pitiless a man stronger in body but weaker in spirit than the unblemished youth of the scene before.

"My God, my God—why hast thou forsaken me?" is perhaps the cry unheard in the fury of the wind that blows away all prayer. God can't possibly hear it through this. There seems to emanate from the central figure a too-late recognition of his frailty and powerlessness in the presence of these surrounding forces.

In the final painting, the winds have died down, and the storm clouds have drifted high over the receding cliffs. The raging rapids from the last scene have emptied into a vast, calm sea: "Old Age." The angel boat is battered, angels' wings broken off. It floats into the shimmering waters, having barely survived the journey.

The boat now carries a somewhat bent old man, hair almost gone, endearingly feeble, looking up to a glorious sight. High in the post-storm sky, a golden light shines toward him, and within it are countless angels. They appear to be lining and guiding the way for the man in his old age to complete his journey to heaven and respite, peace. He returns to an eternal safety and divine love, which have always been there, even in the storm.

In each of these scenes, there is an hourglass attached to the prow of the angel boat, indicating the limited time in the human life. At the end, the hourglass is shattered, indicating not so much death and an ending, but freedom and release into timeless happiness. The suffering and struggling are over. A new peace is begun . . . but . . . Lord, why the journey? Why the tumultuous voyage?

Somehow, we take ownership of what Cole paints in his first two scenes of childhood and youth. We subconsciously sense an entitlement to the idyllic and the comfortable. We hold lovingly to our gentle, nurturing God. We presume and are grateful for heaven's blessings, invincibility, and guardianship when all is going well and we are successful, as in the glow of scene two.

Then life hurts and disappoints us. We send up our cries to God of *why* and *how* and *please.* The same God in whom we trusted puzzles and confuses us when the storms finally turn their fury upon us. We want to keep believing in this ethereal, watchful presence but cry and pound in anguish at its apparent stony silence when we or those we love are left unsaved.

Is it then that our view of life is skewed? We constantly feel in crisis, trying to figure out and explain the problem of evil, suffering, and death—they seem so hateful and hurtful to us. This can carry over to our views of the medical world, where we often get caught up in believing that every single malady or dysfunction should some-how be cured and eliminated. We even strive to eliminate death via life-extending technologies or to eliminate dying by pursuing physician-assisted suicide. In *God, Medicine, and Suffering,* Stanley Hauerwas writes:

> Medicine cannot help but become part of this conspiracy; indeed, now the task of medicine is to go to elaborate lengths to keep us alive, the consequence being that some of us end up being mere physical shells incapable, when we are dying, of knowing we are dying. Because cure, not care, has become medicine's primary purpose, physicians have become warriors engaged in combat with the ultimate adversary—death. Of course, since this is a war that can-not be won, it puts physicians in a peculiar double bind. They must do everything they can to keep us alive, as if living were an end in itself, but then they must endure our blame when, inevitably, they fail. Almost as perplexing is the fact that although doctors are obligated to use every possible medical technology to keep us alive in order to insure that we will die "only when everything possible has

been done," we complain that doctors go to unreasonable lengths to keep us alive.

Your Faith Has Been Your Salvation

It still comes down to the everyday fact that we suffer, individually and collectively. We pray for healing and for peace. We pray for successful surgeries and recoveries from cancers. We pray that someone paralyzed might walk; that a child stricken will be able to live a full, healthy life; that a relationship lost might be regained. We are so often left to wonder if our God hears us. Do prayers really do anything?

Bridget Meehan, in *The Healing Power of Prayer,* gives us her insights:

> Although the healing of sickness can be a sign of salvation, it is not essential that everyone who is saved also be healed of any or all physical or emotional sickness. . . . Healing and suffering are not mutually exclusive. . . . The apostles, like Christ, did not remove all illness or suffering from humankind. . . . Since we are still subject to death and suffering, however, we cannot demand to be liberated from the sources of death, such as sickness and pain. . . . There is no way to know or understand why some people are healed through prayer while others remain ill. . . . No amount of prayer for physical or inner healing will be able to alleviate all our emptiness and struggle.

Though there are many new studies on the power of faith and prayer, these do not *explain* faith and prayer. For those who believe in God, it comes down to a matter of faith. For those who do not believe in God, it must end up being a matter of randomness. For all of us, it remains a mystery. We hear Jesus say many times in the Gospels:

"It is your faith that has healed you" or "Your faith is your salvation." We know also that "because of their lack of faith he could work no miracles there."

The Challenge

The Messiah did not come to get rid of poverty and hunger, of Caesars and their taxes, of death. He came to uplift this poor beggar, to touch this particular leper, to open this man's eyes and this one's ears. He raised this particular Lazarus on this particular day.

What the Messiah came to do for all time was to demonstrate God's love for you. He came to show you how to live within your suffering. He came to demonstrate forgiveness and compassion. Christ died on a cross when he could have avoided death; he suffered when he could have avoided suffering. He showed us by his life on this earth that what we so strenuously seek to avoid is part of what we are to live.

We either believe Jesus, or we don't, when he says, "Today you will be with me in paradise." He also tells us that his father knows exactly what we need. We either walk away sad, as did the rich young man, or we leave behind our perceived security and follow the Lord. We can turn away with the many who could not believe in Jesus, or we can stay with Peter and the apostles, even if in our pained confusion we say merely, "Lord, to whom shall we go?"

God wants you to know that none of your suffering and pain, anguish and loss goes without his notice. He sends himself in others to help you and hold you. When you are alone and unreachable by others, his spirit is within and around you. He hangs on the cross right next to yours; he never leaves your side. He does not run off to save someone else from their death, leaving you abandoned. He does not condemn you because you scream out in pain or cry in anguish. He takes the lashing with you. He stands by your side when you believe you are standing alone, while the world, love, riches, or happiness pass you by.

Yes, it *is* a matter of faith. Even without logical proof we can choose to believe that God is somehow with each suffering individual under every collapsed building, in every torture chamber, in every hospital bed, in every single lonely out-of-the-way place. Jesus can come to you in a tiny piece of bread and in a chalice of wine. God can come to you however he pleases. You can accept the gifts already given you and the manna sent your way each day, or you can blind yourself to the good things in life, blaming God and others for the evil upon which you choose to focus.

In the mystery of this entire journey called life, you are invited to live it to the fullest, including the parts that seem to be so hard. Change the evil that you can change. Endure the pain that you cannot. Share the goodness and the sadness in a spirit that acknowledges that God is there in your midst. Be open to the possibility that you are always part of the miracle. Be open always to the Annie Sullivans, the horse whisperers, the men behind the curtains—to all those the Lord sends. God will reach out to touch your hand and lift you from your pain and loss, even from your anger at him.

Come, pick up your mat, walk with your God.

> *"Can any of you by worrying add a moment to your life-span? If even the smallest things are beyond your control, why are you anxious about the rest? . . . Do not worry anymore. . . . Do not be afraid any longer, little flock, for your Father is pleased to give you the kingdom." (Luke 12:25–26, 29, 32)*

Questions for Your Health

• How can you live out the life you have, despite the pain you have? Even in your pain, weakness, or depression, can you think of ways you are valuable to someone else? Can you think of ways others may need you to help them?

• When you wish your life was how it used to be and not how it has become since the injury or surgery or diagnosis—or simply since getting older—name three things that actually weren't so great before. Then name five ways in which your life is better now, in spite of your burdens. If you can't name five ways, then get busy creating them. It is your only life—stop waiting for someone else to fix it.

• When your doctor says you will just have to live with your pain, that there is nothing else to be done, ask if there are ways he or she can help you live with it: checkups periodically to explore new medicines, referrals for occasional pain-relieving procedures in the event of acute crises, or referrals for alternative care options or psychological support. They are just the people behind the curtain, but it's amazing how a diploma, a medal, or a testimonial can be just what you need. When we have been out searching for witches' broomsticks and lamenting our lack of a brain, a heart, or courage, sometimes it is the small suggestions that help the most.

14

"GO IN PEACE."

The Grace You Have
Been Given

*Peace I leave with you; my peace I give to you. Not as the world gives
do I give it to you. Do not let your hears be troubled or afraid.*

John 14:27

Faith is first a desire to believe and a humility that accepts a lack
of understanding. *Lord, if you will it, you can heal me.* This softness
of the heart nevertheless demands courage. When God says to you,
"Pick up your mat and walk," you may not yet know the way. When
he first says to you, "Your sins are forgiven," you must trust that you
are being freed. Go, therefore, in peace, to love and serve the Lord,
and one another. Two final stories of love:

Mary Ellen

Who was this young woman when she wore dresses and makeup,
tossed her hair playfully? And what was going on now inside the
shaved head, the crescent remnant of a surgeon's blade tracked on
her cropped scalp? Her eyes wandered aimlessly, randomly, vacantly.
No contact could be made with a person behind them. Where did

the tunnels lead when one looked deeply into those large, dark pupils? Her mouth chewed pointlessly. Nutrition entered her system through a tube in her stomach, placed long ago now, as her body had no control over any food or liquid placed in her mouth. Her arms were stuck bent at the elbows, wrists, and fingers, from what are called contractures, the flexor muscles given free reign now that the conscious control centers were no longer in charge. For years she had existed in the nursing home, lying in her bed or propped up and supported in her wheelchair.

She had lived, not died, when her friend's car hit a tree coming home from a high school dance five years before. She now existed in what is medically described as a persistent vegetative state; all "vegetative" functions such as breathing, heartbeat, digestion, and blood filtering worked fine. Only the thin outer layer of her brain didn't work, but that was where all the magic was. That was where all the grade school memories were. That was where her playfulness and charm came from. That was where all her decisions were formed, her actions put in play, her dancing and volleyball set in motion, her knowledge gained. That was where all of *her* came from.

Her physical situation could be described like this: it was as if a car had been left running in perfect working order after the driver had been ejected through a flung-open door. The engine would continue idling until it ran out of gas. In this case, someone kept coming to fill the gas tank, change the oil and filters, and fix whatever seemed to show any problems. Rust was meticulously kept away. Sometimes the car was pushed into the sun, or back into the garage. But it would never be driven again. It was just running, without a driver, without going anywhere.

Such was Mary Ellen, now twenty-three. No miracles had happened. Was Mary Ellen in there anywhere, or was she in limbo, in some celestial holding pattern until her healthy, young body, originally designed to live another seventy years, gave way, stealthily slipping off before anyone had time to race in and rescue her again, as they did that first night by the side of the road, in the emergency room and in the trauma O.R. down the hall?

So, Jesus, is this little girl "only asleep"? Her mother and father have said "talitha koum" a million times, but her eyes merely rove, and her mouth continues to chew. The wailing and the din are long over. In fact, hardly anyone comes around any longer, other than the slow, low-intensity shifts of nurses and caregiving staff. What is her life for now, Lord? Any hints or suggestions? If her family keeps talking to her, playing music, stimulating her, will she wake up? Are they being tested for endurance, like Moses trying to hold his arms aloft over the battlefield so that the armies of Israel would prevail? Aaron had to help, but the book says they won. Is that what this is all about? A test?

One can only do what one can do. So her sheets are meticulously cleaned and kept soft. Her body is cleaned gently and rubbed with oil and skin softener each day. Lambswool padding is placed under all the bony prominences to keep her comfortable and her skin protected. Her digestive system and the basics of bowel and bladder regularity are high on the list of critical tasks in her medical-care plan. Gentle music is played at her bedside, a stuffed animal is placed near her pillow, photographs are hung hopefully within her view—family members and old friends, even pictures of herself as a real, live, walking, talking girl with long hair.

In this world, which our God visited once in person a couple thousand years ago, some very tragic events occur. When faced with the five thousand in need of food, God didn't cure hunger. He asked what the apostles had to give. In Mary Ellen's case, her family members are the ones who give—love and commitment, care and attention, perseverance and courage. They give freely, and others at the nursing home share in those same gifts. The value of life, however damaged and trapped, however mysteriously altered, is affirmed. The miracle, though, is very hard to see through the fog of suffering. Perhaps Mary Ellen is already safe, and it is those who remain who suffer most.

Whatever the degree of "life" we can see in another individual, it is precious in the sight of God, as he showed us in the Gospels. And we, made in the image of God, act for God on this earth. Whether life is born deformed, developmentally damaged, or whether it is altered by trauma, psychological dysfunction, degeneration, or misuse, we are to care for it, with the little it may seem we have. For God, nothing is too great to overcome. When we don't see the happy ending we desire, when we don't even see an end, then it is also hard for us to see God. Perhaps we really only have a part of the vast truth. The care given to those like Mary Ellen is the glimpse of sacrificial love infused throughout the world by the Creator. We are not abandoned. We may be hungry, but the basket is coming around. Look then for what you yourself may share.

Care Is the Cure

A friend's father recently died of pancreatic cancer. It took perhaps three months. No cures came from twenty-first-century medicine. But there was so much healing. I don't think it could have been done any better. As his son said many times, and particularly eloquently at the eulogy during the funeral Mass, this man should have died many times of many things over the last many years. He hadn't. He had actually become healthier, happier, and more full of life the longer he survived his diabetes and cardiovascular disease, his lung dysfunction, and his steroid myopathy.

When the diagnosis of pancreatic cancer was made for this man, his son the doctor knew full well the fate ahead. Aggressive medical treatment was called into action, but the dying process was what became the primary aspect of this person's remaining life. So family and friends put off nearly everything else and arranged time to be together, with father and colleague. Grandchildren had tons of time to frolic around the grand patriarch—and he absolutely delighted in it. That was hard, because it made the leaving that much more bittersweet. He knew he was heading for home but also about to leave the home he had built over a lifetime.

Old misunderstandings were cleared up. Old grudges dismissed. Hurts and wounds were salved and forgiven. Love was brought lavishly to the fore. Prayer was unabashedly part of each day. Gratitude was spoken. Pain was managed and actually wasn't all that bad. Letting go happened, slowly, but steadily and surely, until the final predawn hours when his angel arrived to escort him to his party. His family had to accept that they wouldn't be going to that party until later, and that Dad would be just fine going ahead of them on his own. They all had performed their miracle of overcoming death and sorrow with life and happiness.

As Christ told his disciples when he walked among us, look about you and what do you see? The kingdom of God is at hand. Love one another as I have loved you. *Care* is the cure, the miracle, the healing of a life broken. God has placed eternity in the human mind. He has imbued us with limitless endurance, unfathomable ingenuity, and an indomitable spirit of love, compassion, and hope. Look around you, at all the marvels you see that the human mind has created.

Yes, We Do Have to Live with It—How Will You?

So we have come full circle in this exploration of the circle of pain and suffering talked about at the beginning of the book. Because humanity has the capacity to reflect on itself, we do experience our pains and losses as more than biological events. We do have to live with it all. Because pain ultimately ends up "in our heads," we can sometimes use our minds to help us endure. And not always alone do we have to endure. Because we live in societies and in communities, we suffer together, and we can bear each other's burdens.

Yes, we have anger and frustration. Those are normal reactions, and we can accept them and yet work at moving beyond them. To be sure, we are not always in as much control of our behaviors as we'd like to be. But we must pray to suffer in communion with all those who have suffered before us and with all those who suffer this very moment with us. This does not remove the pain. But in the mystery of thinking beyond the self, all burdens are shared, and somehow perhaps even eased. As we go outside the self, the dominant, all-consuming power of pain is lessened.

We are also given the gifts of one another, allowing us to give and receive comfort and relief. Humanity has developed many miracles through its ingenuity. We can accept whatever help is offered, whatever new drug or therapy, even if it appears not to be nearly enough. The few loaves and fishes fed five thousand. We can learn to live outside the previous perceptions of how help could or could not arrive. From the most modern high-tech microsurgery to the most subtle energy-based healing therapy, we can see and accept Divinity's hand reaching out to touch us from all corners of creation.

Finally, perhaps we can see death as part of life as much as the earth is part of the universe. We can move beyond the gravitational pull of our planet and free ourselves to explore the vastness that is beyond the tiny world in which we live. Likewise, if we can escape the strong ties we have to this life that we know, then certainly we can free ourselves to escape its confines through death and trust in the limitless "eternal" life that awaits us.

Ephphatha—That Is, Be Opened

Ephphatha is the word used by Jesus when he healed a deaf mute. Do you hear Jesus' voice within you, speaking to you, consoling you, encouraging you, calming you? The voice of our God is ever whispering in our hearts and souls. Trust that the divine love constantly seeks to gain access to you. As the Creator's Spirit stirred over the waters of primal earth and brought forth life and abundance and order, so it stirs over, around, and within your own disordered spirit. Do not doubt God's goodness or your own, despite the sadness or pain of your situation.

To assure us of his presence, God came to us in the flesh. He talked with us, walked with us, worked and laughed, cried and suffered with us. He lived the life we live. He lived the life he created. He lived in the world as he found it. God did not cure the world of itself. He did not stop pain and he did not alter time. But he did show us how to live—in love, compassion, and action.

To the leper with a simple, straightforward request and staunchness of faith, he gave dignity, respect, and opportunity to do the great things he desired to accomplish in his life.

To the woman with the hemorrhage, he gave fullness of reconciliation, expiation of guilt, reward for perseverance, and the capacity to boldly stand up before others.

To the man on the mat, he gave recognition amid the passing crowds. God had seen him through all the thirty-eight years he'd lain there, as God sees each of us through all our enduring. He rescued him from a wasted life on a mat. Jesus stepped in where others had not and sent this man off to a bold life of risk and challenge and the opportunity for independence.

To the little girl and her father, Jesus came and created a sacred space, in the middle of all that seemed to have gone wrong. He gave them an explanation. He asked for trust. When the child within each of us is broken, he will come and take us by the hand, saying gently, "Stand up." What if the little girl had died? Countless other little girls and boys no doubt died that very day, that very moment, around the world. Their parents did not get to see them stand up after having "only been asleep." Somehow Jesus must be telling us that all death is only a matter of being "asleep." There is life after this sleep. We can only see the falling. Jesus showed us through his signs and through his own resurrection that there indeed is waking.

To the woman bent over in the bondage of Satan for eighteen years and to the man with the withered hand, Jesus gave compassion and mercy. He tenderly saves those who patiently sacrifice their lives in humility and meekness. He sees the lonely and those who suffer invisibly. He comes to you, even when you have no strength to seek him. He will care for those who are innocently downtrodden, disabled, rejected, ignored, frightened, sacrificed in their accidental births. We must listen to his calls for us to slow down, reach out, lift up, care for, and love.

To the possessed, lost in the disordered tumble of their dysfunctional lives, psyches, addictions, sins, and failings, Jesus said, I am not afraid. You do not scare me off or disgust me. I love you right through your raging to your very core. I see the beauty and the pain in you, and I will embrace you even as you scream, "Leave me alone, Son of God!" You cannot lose me just because you are lost.

To the grateful leper who returned to say thank you, Jesus gave back a life in community and acceptance. To the other nine, he gave the gift of time. Perhaps they were not ready to see their new identities. They had been cured nonetheless. Jesus will give us gifts over and over, desiring that one day we'll realize we are no longer the lepers we believed ourselves to be.

To the hard-hearted, he always gave a chance for reconciliation, and he always gave them their freedom to choose. In ultimate love that risks being rejected, God gives people free will. We must believe that at some moment, in some way, the Creator of all souls gives each soul the choice to accept the invitation to love, in a manner that each soul can clearly understand, and that he gives those chances over and over. No preordained souls are destined to be evil and to die while the rest of us chosen are above the fray. All are chosen; the question is, do all respond to the choosing?

To the dying and to those who lose a loved one to death, life-altering illness, or a destroyed relationship, Jesus says first and foremost, I will die with you. I am with you, I am with him, I am with her in the dying. No one is alone, in this most alone of human experiences. He also says, This is not the end. It is the end, perhaps, to the part that you can see, but it is only the beginning of so much more to come. Why? We cannot answer that. We can only risk believing that God showed up on earth as one of us and specifically told us it would be so. Paradise is waiting. Fear not. Live boldly. Be open to all that is possible, to all that may be unseen, to all that may be difficult to understand.

Remember, each person healed in the Gospels rejoined a world of possible suffering, not a world of no suffering. Each person cured of a disease could get sick again. Each person previously blind and begging, given the miracle of sight, was also given the challenge of living a new life. Each person raised from the dead would one day still die. The thief on the cross saw Christ looking into his eyes, and together they hung there. But they would move on, through that moment of pain.

As for all the sorrow and suffering in the world, we can say that God, who is love, suffers. And thus God shares in our suffering, and somehow that suffering has meaning. Why love with suffering? I suppose Jesus' response would be, "I asked the same question in Gethsemane. Father, I do not wish to drink this cup, but if it is your will, then I will do it. I do not understand it, nor do I want to have to endure the pain and death. But I will give back to you my very life. For you gave it to me, and I trust your love for me is eternal. I let go of me and fall, in love, to you."

In a beautiful song about Abraham and Isaac, titled "God Will Provide a Lamb," the words say that the ram was sent to Abraham to sacrifice instead of his son. It says God will send his Son as a lamb to be offered up instead of us. Sometimes we may hear the words, "Now I need *you* to be the lamb for me. I will share the road of Calvary with you. Your faith will be your salvation."

The Road Ahead

Each time I look down the road ahead
I look for goodness there for me.
What will become of me after this night?
Is there a dawn ahead for me?

Each day brings its newness
And with each moment
I'm more aware
I shall go on
And live each day.

Come to me and I'll renew you
Enter into me
And be born
Until you die
You shall not live.

Break your body first
And spill your blood
Then you will come to know
The cost of freeing men
And through your death
Men shall be free.

Each time I look down the road ahead
I look for goodness there for me
What will become of me after this night
Is there a dawn ahead for me?

Chris Murphy, *Strings 'n Things*, 1975

The Final Discourse

Do you realize what I have done for you? . . . If I, therefore, the master and teacher, have washed your feet, you ought to wash one another's feet. . . .

I give you a new commandment: love one another. As I have loved you, so you also should love one another. This is how all will know that you are my disciples, if you have love for one another.

Do not let your hearts be troubled. . . . I am the way and the truth and the life. . . . Amen, amen, I say to you, whoever believes in me will do the works that I do, and will do greater ones than these. . . .

Remember the word I spoke to you, "No slave is greater than his master." . . .

Amen, amen, I say to you, you will weep and mourn, while the world rejoices; you will grieve, but your grief will become joy. When a woman is in labor, she is in anguish because her hour has arrived; but when she has given birth to a child, she no longer remembers the pain because of her joy that a child has been born into the world. So you also are now in anguish. But I will see you again, and your hearts will rejoice, and no one will take your joy away from you. On that day you will not question me about anything. . . .

In the world you will have trouble, but take courage, I have conquered the world. (John 13:12, 14, 34–35; 14:1, 6, 12; 15:20; 16:20–23, 33)

AFTERWORD

This book was not intended to be a how-to for pain management itself. It was a reflective and contemplative effort at learning from the words and actions of our Lord in his earthly encounters with people in pain and how we might gain comfort and insight into present-day dealings with our pain or the pain suffered by the people we know and love.

Medical answers for the practical day-to-day treatment and management of pain would require a separate book. Yet, let me leave you with some words from my medical mind, following upon the body of my book from my spiritual heart.

Everyone experiences pain via that fourth circle of suffering (touched on in the sidebar of chapter 2) in unique ways dependent on specific situations.

Acute pain is a biologic warning or indication of an injury or a dysfunction to which the body wants to call attention. Most acute pain is self-limited and can be resolved with a little rubbing, soothing, hugging, ice, and time. Simple over-the-counter medicines such as aspirin, acetaminophen, or anti-inflammatories are the mainstays of the vast majority of minor to moderate pain events. Alternative medicine—herbal or topical substances—are the options for many people.

Physical hands-on treatments are critical to the successful treatment of many pain and injury problems. Physical therapy is my most utilized area of expertise in this area of pain management. I am very demanding in finding good therapists who do more than just apply simple heating devices or cold packs, who do more than just watch three people at a time do exercises that could be done just as easily at home. A good physical therapist is a medical detective, attempting to discern the biomechanical causes of injury, strain, and pain, and then seeking to relieve immediate pain while working on prevention of future recurrent injury and pain.

Other hands-on professionals include occupational therapists, chiropractors, naprapaths, massage therapists, and therapeutic body workers (or Rolfers). There are more practitioners in energy work, therapeutic touch, and other mind–body approaches. Specific exercise approaches such as Pilates, Feldenkrais, and Alexander are valuable in treating certain disorders. Specific techniques such as McKenzie, craniosacral, muscle energy, and myofascial therapies should be put into use appropriately by skilled therapists for conditions such as disc injuries, headaches, muscle strains, and chronic pain, to name just a few.

Acupuncture is an entire system of care. Saying that you received some acupuncture would be like a person in the middle of China saying that he or she received some American medicine. That could mean pills, surgery, scans, and therapies. Acupuncture, though we see it as merely getting some needles placed around the body, is a multidimensional system of care with a history of over five thousand years. Does it replace surgery, antibiotics, physical therapy, or other Western approaches? No. That is why approaches such as acupuncture are now referred to as "complementary" practices rather than "alternative."

Regarding Western medicine, do not be intimidated by taking strong pain medicine, with the proper safeguards; neither be cavalier about it nor allow yourself to believe you are totally dependent on it. Opiates are as old as nature. These are the morphinelike drugs, and there are many available. They can be abused, as in the use of heroin on the street or in the misuse of prescription medicines such as the more commonly known Vicodin and OxyContin™. These are good medicines. I frequently prescribe them. Yet they must be respected and controlled. There are many brands of pain medicines, from tablets, liquids, and suckers to patches or injections. For serious chronic-pain patients who have endured failed surgeries and other various treatments, pumps can be implanted in the spinal canal to deliver morphine more effectively, or tiny electrode strips, called a dorsal column stimulator, can be placed along the spinal cord to block certain pain signals.

The point is, there are many, many effective approaches to pain management. Some can be so effective that patients consider them miraculous. On the other hand, some patients and their pain can be so recalcitrant that it seems nothing works, or nothing is tolerated. Sometimes such pain is what is called centralized and is thought to be caught deep within the circuitry of the spinal cord and brain, thus not reachable by medicines and procedures available so far. Remember the stories of the miracles: many people had to wait for years before Jesus showed up in their lives. Many people today will have to wait through pain until new approaches are discovered which might work better for them. Yes, they will live with their pain. How to live with pain was much of the purpose behind the reflections in this book.

On the other hand, we must take advantage of support and skills available right now to help us live with pain that medicines and surgeries cannot erase. I have mentioned them before; you must allow yourself to learn from psychologists and other experts in the mental and emotional aspects of pain. You must look with a critical eye at your own personality, habits, and entrenched ways of thinking and ask yourself how they may be contributing to the vicious circle of chronic, unremitting pain. You must take on the work of self-examination, must take responsibility for battling for your life. Meditation, yoga, tai chi, qigong, self-hypnosis, and biofeedback are just a few of the self-help techniques available.

Finally, there is prayer. Reflect on the sacred stories and on the words of God. Give yourself time to quiet down and listen. Risk hearing what you don't want to hear. Risk hearing what seems to be nothing for a while. God may want you to just sit within his power and grace. It is like sitting on the beach to rest an aching, tired body.

The sand supports you. The sun warms you. The tan just happens. God supports you and warms you. The healing can happen if you are open to God's way of healing you, and not just to the way you are demanding that healing occur.

God has placed the miracles of his work all around you, in the people he has created to be on this earth the same time you are here. Do not ignore their abilities to help you. Remember that many people did not recognize God in the carpenter's son and so missed the most wonderful encounter they ever could have asked for. God is present in the people around you, both in their being and their skills. And he is present in the unlimited power of his grace placed within you. Rise up, pick up your mat, and walk. Your faith will heal you.

WORKS CITED

Dossey, Larry. *Healing Words: The Power of Prayer and the Practice of Medicine*. New York: HarperCollins, 1993.

_____. *Prayer Is Good Medicine: How to Reap the Healing Benefits of Prayer*. New York: HarperCollins, 1996.

Hall, Douglas John. *God & Human Suffering: An Exercise in the Theology of the Cross*. Minneapolis, Minn.: Augsberg Publishing House, 1986.

Hauerwas, Stanley. *God, Medicine, and Suffering*. Grand Rapids, Mich.: William B. Eerdmans, 1990.

Kennedy, Eugene C. *The Pain of Being Human*. New York: The Crossroad Publishing Company, 1997.

Kushner, Harold S. *When Bad Things Happen to Good People*. New York: Avon Books, 1981.

Meehan, Bridget. *The Healing Power of Prayer*. Ligouri, Mo.: Ligouri Publications, 1988.

Morris, David B. *The Culture of Pain*. Berkeley, Calif.: University of California Press, 1991.

_____. *Illness and Culture in the Postmodern Age*. Berkeley, Calif.: University of California Press, 1998.

Neuhaus, Richard John. *Death on a Friday Afternoon: Meditations on the Last Words of Jesus from the Cross*. New York: Basic Books, 2000.

Wolterstorff, Nicholas. *Lament for a Son*. Grand Rapids, Mich.: William B. Eerdmans, 1987.

A Special Invitation

Loyola Press invites you to become one of our Loyola Press Advisors! Join our unique online community of people willing to share with us their thoughts and ideas about Catholic life and faith. By sharing your perspective, you will help us improve our books and serve the greater Catholic community.

From time to time, registered advisors are invited to participate in online surveys and discussion groups. Most surveys will take less than ten minutes to complete. Loyola Press will recognize your time and efforts with gift certificates and prizes. Your personal information will be held in strict confidence. Your participation will be for research purposes only, and at no time will we try to sell you anything.

Please consider this opportunity to help Loyola Press improve our products and better serve you and the Catholic community. To learn more or to join, visit **www.SpiritedTalk.org** and register today.

—*The Loyola Press Advisory Team*